**DATE DUE**

| | | | |
|---|---|---|---|
| | | | |
| | | | |
| | | | |
| | | | |
| | | | |
| | | | |
| | | | |
| | | | |
| | | | |
| | | | |
| | | | |

**LACKAWANNA COUNTY
LIBRARY SYSTEM**
520 VINE STREET
SCRANTON, PA
18509

DEMCO

Sounds
of
Healing

# Sounds
## of
# Healing

**A Physician Reveals the**

**Therapeutic Power of**

**Sound, Voice, and Music**

MITCHELL L. GAYNOR, M.D.

BROADWAY BOOKS   NEW YORK

**BROADWAY**

Broadway Books titles may be purchased for business or promotional use or for special sales. For information, please write to: Special Markets Department, Random House, Inc., 1540 Broadway, New York, NY 10036.

BROADWAY BOOKS and its logo, a letter B bisected on the diagonal, are trademarks of Broadway Books, a division of Random House, Inc.

Visit our website at www.broadwaybooks.com

Essence and Energetic Re-creation are proprietary marks of Dr. Mitchell Gaynor for stress reduction and meditation.

*Library of Congress Cataloging-in-Publication Data*
   Gaynor, Mitchell L., 1956–
     Sounds of healing: a physician reveals
the therapeutic power of sound, voice,
and music / by Mitchell L. Gaynor.
       p.   cm.
   Includes bibliographical references and index.
   ISBN 0-7679-0265-3 (hardcover)
   1. Music therapy.  2. Holistic medicine .  I. Title.
   ML3920.G22   1999
   615.8′ 5154—dc21               99-17241
                             CIP

FIRST EDITION

Designed by Lee Fukui

99  00  01  02  03  10  9  8  7  6  5  4  3  2

The author acknowledges permission to reprint the following:

Excerpt from "What Is Toning and How Do You Do It?" in *The Healing Voice* by Joy Gardner-Gordon. Copyright © 1993. Reprinted with permission from The Crossing Press, P.O. Box 1048, Freedom, CA, 95019.

Excerpt adapted with permission of Sterling Publishing Co., Inc., 387 Park Avenue South, New York, NY, 10016, from *Healing Imagery & Music* by Carol A. Bush, copyright © 1995 by Carol A. Bush.

Excerpt from *The Music Within You* by Shelley Katsh and Carol Merle-Fishman. Copyright © Barcelona Publishers, 1998. Reprinted by permission of Barcelona Publishers, 4 Whitebrook Road, Gilsum, NH 03448.

Excerpts from *Your Sixth Sense* by Belleruth Naparstek © 1997, by Belleruth Naparstek. Reprinted by permission of HarperCollins Publishers, Inc.

Excerpt taken from *Infinite Happiness*, written by Masami Saionji. Copyright © 1996, by Masami Saionji. Used by permission of Element Books, Inc., Boston, MA.

*To the Children of Tibet*

## DISCLAIMER

The patients whose stories I've told in this book have given me consent to use their clinical histories. To protect their privacy, I have changed names, transposed events, merged the stories of different people, and altered identifying characteristics. The techniques described in this book are no substitutes for professional care. Because everyone is different, a physician must diagnose individual conditions and supervise all health problems. I urge you to seek out the best medical resources available to help you make informed decisions.

# Contents

# Acknowledgments

I would like first and foremost to acknowledge my wife, Cathy, for her ever-present love and encouragement. Thank you, as well, to Ron Young and my father for their tireless support of this work. I am also indebted to Deborah Chiel for her invaluable creative input and editorial assistance; without her, this book could not have been written. My agent, Janis Vallely, has been unfailingly encouraging, insightful, and wise in her shepherding of this project from concept to fruition. Thank you to the superb team of individuals at Broadway Books who have labored with me to make this book a reality: Bill Shinker, Lauren Marino, Ann Campbell, Trigg Robinson, and Jennifer Swihart. I am also very grateful to Janet Goldstein, who heard the sound of the crystal bowls and had the vision to acquire the book. Many thanks to Kitty Farmer for her tireless efforts orchestrating my lecture tour, and to Tracey Donner for her invaluable public relations skills. Special thanks are in order to all the physicians and staff at the Strang Cancer Prevention Center whose commitment to the scientific study of holistic medicine and nutrition remains steadfast.

The following individuals were also very generous with their time and expertise in the area of sound, music, and mind-body healing: Bracha Adrezin; Phoebe Atkinson; Joseph-Mark Cohen; Shulamith Elson; Steven Halpern; Shelley Katsh, C.M.T.–B.C., C.S.W.; Govindha McRostie, O.M.D., N.D.; Hollis Melton; Jim Oliver; Con Potanin, M.D.; Jill Purce; Mark Rider, Ph.D.; Linda Rodgers, C.S.W.; Bri. Maya Tiwari; Jeffrey Thompson, D.C.; and Alicia Trombla. A special thanks to Henry Dreher, who unstintingly shared his time and knowledge of the mind-body field.

I would also like to thank those teachers who have facilitated my own growth and abilities as a physician-healer: Dr. Larry Dossy, Dr. Robert Jaffe, Pir Vilayat Inayat Khan, Fran Richey, Shyalpa Rinpoche, Jack Steiman, and Masayoshi Yamaguchi.

# The Singing Bowls

In 1991, I was asked by another attending physician at New York Hospital to evaluate a new patient in the Intensive Care Unit. I was immediately drawn to Ödsal, a Tibetan monk in his late thirties, a gentle, soft-spoken man, whose warmth and humility were tinged with a sense of sorrowful stoicism. Ödsal had a rare disease called cardiomyopathy, an enlargement of the heart that normally results in congestive heart failure. As is typical of people with this life-threatening ailment, he had developed progressive anemia and was extremely ill. He urgently needed a heart transplant but was having no success finding a match.

Having been brought in for a hematology consultation, I proceeded to conduct a battery of tests and started him on the appropriate drug regimen to combat his anemia. Because I subscribe to the belief—well researched by mind-body scientists—that what happens to us on the emotional and spiritual levels affects us physiologically, I asked Ödsal to tell me something about his background and how he had grown up.

He explained that he had fled his native Tibet as a young child with his parents and brother after the Chinese invaded his country in 1950. He vividly recalled the searing sense of dislocation and

1

poverty that he and his family experienced as exiles in India. The family lived a hand-to-mouth existence; there was barely enough money for food. When he was three years old, his parents decided to leave him and his brother at an orphanage rather than watch the two children starve to death. All these years later, his pain was still fresh when he described his feelings of abandonment, how he called out to his mother and father as they said good-bye and walked away.

The orphanage was run by Tibetan monks who raised him to be a monk, educating him in the Buddhist religion and Tibetan culture. He was also an extraordinary artist whose drawings of mandalas impressed me with their intricacy and beauty. But his heart had been forever shattered from the grief of separation from his parents, who could afford to visit him only once a year. Each time they left, he said, he felt his anguish as sharply as if he were experiencing it for the very first time.

His suffering was compounded by an overwhelming sense of hopelessness that his country would ever free itself of China's brutal domination. I began to see that his stoicism stemmed from a place of dark despair; it was not the stoicism of detachment that the Buddhists try to cultivate but rather one of deep pessimism about the future of Tibet.

My initial sense upon meeting Ödsal was that his severe heart condition was, to some degree, a physical manifestation of an equally acute state of psychic distress. His life story bore out my impression. I could address the physical symptoms: Ödsal responded well to the medication and was soon feeling strong enough that he was able to leave the hospital. But I knew that Ödsal's disease ran much deeper, that he was literally suffering from a broken heart. My medical intervention, useful as it was, could not heal his underlying wound.

Because he was a Tibetan monk who had spent his life in meditation, I felt it would be presumptuous of me to undertake the kind of healing work I'd been doing with my other patients.

Nevertheless, I spent a great deal of time talking to him about his childhood experiences and expressing my care in whatever way I could. Then one of my colleagues told Ödsal about my ESSENCE Guided Imagery, and Ödsal asked me to teach him the technique. Although I felt somewhat insecure about explaining guided imagery techniques to a monk who had spent his life practicing meditation, I reluctantly agreed. Ödsal liked the imagery, which was very different from the kind of meditation he was used to practicing, and I could feel a lessening of the burden of sadness he had carried since childhood.

The next week, when he came to my office for a follow-up visit, he brought me a Tibetan dahl, a metal cylinder similar to a bell. I was deeply touched by his unexpected and generous gift and very taken by the sound it produced. I had already begun to study various Eastern and Western spiritual practices, so I asked Ödsal whether he would teach me some of the sacred Tibetan chants he had learned as a youngster at the monastery. He agreed to come to my apartment several days later, and when he arrived, I saw that he had brought with him a Tibetan singing bowl of the sort that the monks of his lineage commonly used to accompany their chanting and meditation.

We removed our shoes and settled ourselves cross-legged on the living room floor. Ödsal took out a small wooden baton and moved it lightly around the rim of the bowl, in much the same way that you might trace the lip of a wineglass with your finger. The clamor of the New York City streets, so audible outside my window, fell away as the eerie, otherworldly tones of the bowl filled the space around us. The sound—a rich, deep note with a strong vibrato that resembled nothing I had ever heard before—was so exhilarating that tears of joy sprang to my eyes. I could feel the vibration physically resonating through my body, touching my core in such a way that I felt in harmony with the universe. I did not, at that moment, make a conscious decision to further explore the singing bowls. It was almost as if I didn't have a choice in the matter, because I immediately intuited that playing the bowls would change my life, and the lives of many of my patients.

## BEYOND MEDICAL SCHOOL:
## A DOCTOR'S AWAKENING

If somebody had told me when I was a medical student in Dallas, Texas, that one day I would be teaching my patients to use singing bowls to heal themselves, I would have thought he or she was crazy. Yet today, only fifteen years later, prominently displayed in my consultation room at the renowned Strang Cancer Prevention Center, where I am Director of Oncology and Integrative Medicine, is a beautiful ten-inch quartz crystal bowl, which plays a key role in my busy practice of oncology and internal medicine. Although I once prescribed only the traditional remedies for the treatment of cancer and other ailments, I no longer see a contradiction between chanting and chemotherapy, between visualization and radiation. In fact, just the opposite: I openly advocate for what has come to be known as holistic medicine—combining allopathic regimens with complementary therapies that include nutritional supplements of herbs and algae as well as regular visits to acupuncturists and energy healers. You'll notice that I refer to these modalities as "complementary," rather than "alternative." I have long since come to accept nontraditional, holistic approaches as necessities, rather than potential options, that must be integrated with the care and treatment of my patients.

Given my rather innovative paradigm for healing, some might label me a bit unconventional. I assure you that one doesn't necessarily follow the other. I attended the University of Texas–Southwestern Medical School, one of the most rigorous and competitive institutions in the country, where class rankings and grade point averages are figured to the *thousandth* of a decimal point. I did well enough there that when I graduated I was accepted as an intern at New York Hospital, the prestigious teaching hospital affiliated with Cornell University Medical School, where I eventually became a clinical fellow in hematology and oncology. I later spent a year as a postdoctoral fellow in molecular biology at Rockefeller University, then completed my training with an appointment at New York Hospital as the chief medical resident. In other words, I had the best possible educational foundation in Western medicine, one that gave me a rock-solid grounding in all the state-of-the-art lifesaving techniques that medical science has to offer in this last decade of the twentieth century.

But something was missing—the amalgam of psychology and spirituality that would satisfy my patients' needs to be treated as whole human beings. I first felt this void as a medical student, eager to absorb every lesson our instructors had to offer. At the busy county hospital where I did my rotations, the patients were the occasional butt of jokes among the medical staff. Perhaps the humor was a necessary antidote to the life-or-death demands of the job, but it reinforced for me the sense that we students were being taught to divorce ourselves from our emotions. We were often reprimanded for talking too long to patients. We were criticized for feeling sad or sympathetic because we were "getting too involved." We were rewarded, on the other hand, for being fast and efficient, for treating and releasing patients as quickly as possible, for walling ourselves off from our hearts.

If this absence of feeling was the model for my medical school experience, it was even more the prevailing ethos during my internship and residency. The emphasis was placed almost exclusively on information and knowledge: How many papers could we quote from? Did we have the most up-to-date facts and figures memorized and ready to spit out on command? Could we cite the latest set of statistics on any given study?

No one ever urged us to empathize with our patients. The men and women we treated were seen as cases, rather than human beings. Never mind that they brought with them the totality of their life experiences—all their anguish and joy, fear and hope, past traumas and future ambitions. We were discouraged from considering the possible underlying causes of disease, other than proven cause-and-effect links such as family history, disease pathogens, or environmental factors. We were to concern ourselves only with the symptoms, diagnosis, and medical treatment of whatever illness had landed them in their hospital bed.

Every day I struggled with a medical culture that insisted I keep my distance from patients, and my inclination to get more deeply involved with them. Perhaps my perspective was skewed because as a young child, I had watched my mother die of cancer. I knew about pain and loss. I knew about the will to live, the impulse to keep on fighting to survive, the need to surrender and grieve when every viable medical intervention has been exhausted. I wanted to know more about the people I was treating: What mattered to them? What were they about? Who were they beyond their most obvious identity as "cancer patient"?

In college I had developed an interest in world religions and philosophy. I had also begun to meditate on an almost daily basis. Through meditation, I had learned to take deep breaths and stay calm when I was studying for finals or writing papers. The practice had also improved my ability to concentrate. On a deeper level, meditation had given me treasured moments of realization that I was part of, rather than alone in, the universe—a comforting recognition for a college student who was away from home for the first time and living in a much bigger city than Plainview, the small town in northwestern Texas where I had spent my childhood.

The time constraints of medical school and my postgraduate studies had forced me to give up this practice, but I knew from firsthand experience that meditation was, at the very least, soothing and relaxing. Yet my esteemed physician-professors never recommended the use of relaxation techniques and meditation, which studies had proven could help alleviate many of the worst side effects of chemotherapy, including anticipatory nausea and vomiting.

I remember my frustration verging on despair as time and again one of the more seasoned oncologists under whom I did my postresidency training delivered the cold-blooded diagnosis of, for example, lung cancer: "You'll very likely experience hair loss, nausea, vomiting, and/or fatigue. You will also probably need a blood transfusion. The statistics tell us that most people live three to four months with your type of cancer. I'll see you in two weeks to start chemotherapy."

It was incredible to me that these brilliant and highly skilled physicians seemed to screen out their patients' inevitable reactions of devastation and bewilderment after hearing such news. The cancer diagnosis was terrifying enough. Now they also had to anticipate treatments that promised potentially punishing side effects and an uncertain future. Yet nothing was being offered to relieve their stress or pain. Nor was there nearly enough kindness on the part of the doctors who—from their patients' perspective—suddenly seemed to hold in their hands all the power to heal and give life. I realized, even then, that in the midst of so many discussions about radiation, chemo regimens, and bone marrow transplants, many deeper, perhaps more subtle words were left unspoken.

I will never forget one patient I met while I was in medical school, an orthopedic surgeon who had metastatic lung cancer (i.e., the cancer had spread beyond the primary tumor to other parts of the body). Opinionated and imperious, he clearly reveled in the authority conferred on him by his medical degree. Now, suddenly, the tables had been turned. This stern, headstrong man lay helpless and scared in the hospital bed, desperately searching his doctors' faces for signs of reassurance and hope. He wept uncontrollably, hardly able to believe that such a fate could befall him. "Why is this happening to me?" he asked repeatedly. "What did I do to deserve this?"

His agonizing questions echoed those put to me by many other patients. The common motif was the distorted assumption that they did indeed deserve their disease; they must have committed some terrible wrong or hurt someone badly, to be so cruelly punished. The therapists and psychiatrists who visited them in the hospital tried to help, but they usually focused on the more obvious problems: Who would take care of their family? Were they worried about how they'd look after they lost their hair? Certainly, these were matters worth talking about, but even these mental health professionals were sidestepping any real investigation into the deeper realms of the psyche or spirit.

I like to think that I brought a broader, more open-minded approach to alleviating my patients' emotional anguish. I tried to listen when they talked about their grief and fear. I made a concerted effort to give them the warmth and sensitivity they so plainly needed. But I cannot take credit for deciding to teach them about meditation, visualization, and other relaxation techniques. Quite the contrary. It was my patients who taught me to believe in and trust these methods.

## KEYS TO REMARKABLE RECOVERIES

I began taking note of patients who appeared to be experiencing miraculous recoveries. One woman I treated when I was first in private practice had metastatic breast cancer and appeared to be very close to death. Donna's face was pale and ashen-colored, and she was so weak that she could hardly walk. Some weeks after our initial consultation, she appeared at my office wearing lipstick and looking wonderful. Her color had greatly improved, as had her spirits. I was amazed by the difference and asked what she had done to effect such a change. "I went to see an energy healer," she replied. Although I pressed her for details, she couldn't give me any insights into his work. The outcome was obvious, however. Donna was getting better with each passing week.

Perhaps it's because she believes in him, I told myself. Maybe that's how and why the healing had been accomplished.

Soon thereafter, a patient was referred to me who had metastatic lung cancer. A Vietnam War pilot who had been awarded both the Silver Star and Purple Heart, Charles had been through every conceivable cancer therapy, but none of them had stopped the growth of his cancer. He was now so sick that he was confined to bed. I advised his wife to arrange for him to be admitted to a hospice for the terminally ill. And then, inexplicably, Charles's condition seemed to reverse itself. Not only was he not dying, but the growth of his metastatic tumors came to a standstill. Charles soon began to feel strong enough to leave his bed and begin to participate again in his normal routines. Soon he was ready to resume his chemotherapy, and not long after that, he went back to work.

Once again astonished by the transformation, I sought an explanation for this apparent miracle. "You're not going to believe this," Charles said sheepishly. "My wife called in a healer." Although I hadn't expected Charles to survive much longer than a week or two, he lived for four more years, all the while continuing to work with his healer.

My curiosity had been piqued by Donna and Charles, and I asked their permission to call the people who had treated them. As far back as medical school, I had sensed that sick people might be able to use their illness as an opportunity to learn profound lessons about their lives. Donna's and Charles's healers, and others I subsequently spoke to, validated my belief. They all spoke of shifting our perspective from the tight grip of anxiety, self-pity, and guilt, toward a fuller experience of the authentic self.

Persuaded by their thinking, I rekindled my interest in Eastern philosophies and began again to find time to meditate, if only for twenty or so minutes a day. Then, through yet another of my patients, I had the great fortune to meet a truly gifted healer, Masayoshi Yamaguchi, a Qi Gong master and former musician. I was introduced to him by a Japanese woman, Hiroko, who had a hereditary form of colon cancer that had metastasized to her liver. She had previously been told by two oncologists that she had no more than a month or two to live. All they could offer her at this point, they both said, was a prescription for round-the-clock morphine to ease her pain until the cancer completed its inevitable course and her systems stopped functioning.

Hiroko, whose husband was a wealthy businessman, had traveled from Japan to consult with me. If I had based my judgment solely on her records, I no doubt would have agreed with my Japanese colleagues. But something amazing and wonderful appeared to be taking place. Hiroko was making slow but steady progress back to health. When she came to my office, she was already well enough to begin a course of chemotherapy in order to decrease the size of the tumor and alleviate her pain.

I could attribute Hiroko's improvement only to the fact that she was being treated by Yamaguchi, who spent one week a month with her in New York. During our many conversations, Yamaguchi explained his work as a combination of deep breathing, meditation, Tai Chi, guided imagery, and movement that focused on learning how to direct a person's life energy throughout the body in order to enhance health and well-being. I soon began incorporating his ideas in my medical practice. The results were nothing short of remarkable.

Patients whose illnesses normally would have debilitated them were able to spend quality time with their families and go to work on a regular basis. There were also those who were able to make significant psychological and spiritual breakthroughs that enabled them to live much longer than medical statistics would have predicted. Hiroko was one such patient; thanks to Yamaguchi's ministrations and methods, she survived for three years with a cancer that would otherwise have killed her in four weeks.

## ÖDSAL AND THE SINGING BOWLS

I began searching for healing modalities that could tangibly and reliably help my patients to achieve these transformations. A turning point in my search occurred when I met Ödsal. My initial exposure to the sound of the singing bowls was so thrilling that I wanted to learn all I could about them. Ödsal took me to a store that specialized in Tibetan wares and helped me pick out several bowls, one or more of which I began playing every morning as part of my daily meditation practice. In a surprisingly short time, I found that I was much less vulnerable to stress than I had been in the past. I could more easily avoid conflicts, as well as the minor irritations that once would have made me lose my temper.

I found in Ödsal a remarkable role model and example—a human being who never stopped giving or teaching, who was always more concerned about the needs of others than his own. Even when he was very ill, it was his pleasure to make gifts of his professional-quality portraits and drawings to nurses, doctors, and anyone else who happened to visit him.

I felt myself becoming more compassionate toward all the people in my life and more intuitive about my patients' emotional needs and medical conditions. They seemed to welcome the opportunity for a relationship with a doctor that was as much about empathetic support as the latest advances in medical procedures. I had already been urging my patients to use guided imagery, meditation, deep relaxation exercises, and a nutritionally sound dietary regimen, all of which were integral components of my holistic approach to cancer and other illnesses. Now, the singing bowls became a door through which I could enter an entirely new realm: the healing effects of sound and music.

As I continued my readings in Eastern religions, I was inspired to study with Pir Vilayat Inayat Khan, the head of the Sufi Order in the West, whose father, Hazrat Inayat Khan, brought the message of this obscure mystical Islamic sect to the United States at the beginning of the twentieth century. Hazrat Inayat Khan was already a highly acclaimed musician in India when his spiritual master chose him to spread the Sufi teachings throughout the West. "Fare forth . . . and tune the hearts of men to the divine harmony," his guru instructed him. Hazrat Inayat Khan left behind a legacy of prescient, poetic writings about the human spirit, our connection to the cosmos, and how we can use sound and breath to promote health and healing.

An important element in Sufism is its emphasis on deep breathing and chanting; indeed, the Sufi expression for sound and music, *ghiza-i-ruh,* means "food for the soul." Chanting the vowels in such a way as to hear the harmonics—the mixture of tones beyond the fundamental or dominant tone that is produced when we sing or strike a note on a musical instrument—is an intrinsic part of Sufi ritual. Indeed, Pir Vilayat has said that "the true healing power of sound" comes from the chanting of harmonics.

The Russian philosopher G. I. Gurdjieff used the word *essence* to describe that which is our truest self or soul. I have come to understand the term to mean the infinite, immutable, borderless self that is both whole by itself, and integrated and whole in society and the universe.

Many Eastern spiritual and Western philosophical schools identify a similar spiritual state of being—whether referred to as Atman, Brahman, unity consciousness, unconditioned awareness, or transcendent self—in which we no longer identify with "emotions," "mind," "self," or any circumscribed mental or physical reality. We move to a transpersonal plane in which we are at one with others and the universe or the "Absolute," and the self as a separate entity is dissolved. This does not mean we become fuzzy-headed or float into outer space; indeed, the paradox is that we can remain entirely grounded when we realize our essence.

The more committed I became to playing the singing bowls, the more I began to feel my "essential" self resonating with my surroundings, my family, and the people with whom I came into contact. The results were even more profound when I added another element, the chanting of the vowel sounds that I had read about in Sufi and other Eastern literatures.

The famous story is told about French physician Alfred Tomatis, M.D., who has been recognized by the French Academies of Science and Medicine for his revolutionary research and clinical work in the area of hearing and sound. In the late 1960s, at a Benedictine monastery in the South of France, many of the monks were suffering from what appeared to be a rare and undiagnosable illness. They were inexplicably exhausted, unable to perform their normal tasks. Yet none of the doctors who had previously been consulted could shed any light on what might be the cause of this mysterious epidemic of fatigue. Indeed, one suggestion—that the brothers abandon their habitual vegetarian diet and begin to eat meat—only exacerbated the situation.

Tomatis was invited to the monastery, and his opinion was sought regarding their ailment. As he described it, "seventy of the ninety monks were slumping in their cells like wet dishrags." After examining the men and taking their histories, he discovered what he believed to be the source of the problem. In the wake of the Vatican II reforms authorized by the Catholic Church in the mid-'60s, a young abbot, newly arrived at the monastery, had decreed that the brothers should abandon their traditional practice of singing Gregorian chants six to eight hours each day and instead use the time for more meaningful pursuits. Tomatis, who has been called "the Einstein of sound," immediately surmised that the chanting had functioned as a way to energize the monks by "awakening the field of [their] consciousness." He suggested that they recommence chanting; within five months the brothers were fully recovered from their lassitude and had resumed their regular routine, which included only a very few hours of sleep.

Tomatis describes the Gregorian chants—with their simple melody lines, absence of tempo, and emphasis on long, slow breaths—as "fantastic energy food." Clearly, the chanting provided spiritual and emotional nourishment to the monks, who lived otherwise spartan, unadorned lives. As I read Tomatis's account of his experience, I thought of my patients. They were having to endure demanding, sometimes painful, and always anxiety-provoking encounters with mainstream medicine, encounters that frequently involved stays in hospitals that are themselves spartan institutions. Without some form of spiritual sustenance, people who confront cancer and other serious illness often feel isolated, confused, fearful, forced to fend for themselves. Indeed, I had seen more than a few patients slumped apathetically in my waiting room or in their hospital beds, their affect reminiscent of Tomatis's description of the monks before he restored emotional energy food to their daily diet.

I wanted to find a source of sustenance for my patients, but I couldn't expect them to master the art of Gregorian chanting, which requires a minimum of four years of single-minded dedication and training. A more practical solution presented itself in the *bija* mantras, the seven single-syllable Sanskrit words that correspond to the seven chakras—energy centers in the body—an intrinsic part of Hindu, Sufi, and other Eastern philosophies.

The Sufis assign particular divine attributes to the vowels, each of which corresponds to a chakra—or energy center—in the body, as follows:

LAM—the root (the area of the groin)

VAM—the belly (between the navel and pubic bone)

RAM—the solar plexus

YAM—the heart

HAM—the throat

OM—between the eyebrows (also known as the third eye)

ALL SOUND (encompasses all the sound frequencies in nature)—the crown (Many spiritual masters believe this is the
spot from which the soul enters and leaves the body.)

These mantras, which are commonly used during silent
meditations, are fundamental sounds that help to focus and calm
the mind. Because they are both easy to pronounce and to remember, they would serve as an excellent introduction to the
process of chanting in tune with the bowls. I next began experimenting with the sounds, expanding the possible combinations
of vowels and syllables into a longer list of "mantra sounds" from
which my patients and I could create what I began to think of as
our personal and unique life songs.

As I developed these sound techniques through my own
practice and taught them to my patients, I came to the startling
realization that I could help them achieve in only a few sessions
shifts in perspective that normally took a year or two to accomplish with relaxation techniques that did not include sound. Here
were people undergoing the rigors of cancer treatment, who
were nevertheless able to focus on a creative and joyous process
that removed them from the relentless anticipation of physical
pain and emotional distress. They were finding new ways to
express and transcend their deepest selves. They were literally
finding their "own song to sing," to borrow a phrase from cancer
psychotherapist Lawrence LeShan, Ph.D., in the midst of grueling
medical treatments.

I recall one woman I treated for fibromyalgia, a difficult-to-
treat disorder characterized by chronic pain in different parts of
the body. Anita, an accountant in her early forties, suffered from
severe discomfort in her shoulder and arms, and standard
painkillers were almost completely ineffective. She was reluctant
when I first suggested that she try chanting and playing a bowl in
order to relieve her pain. "It's not my kind of thing," she flatly declared when I made the suggestion. Besides, she informed me, her

family had always made fun of her for her "tin ear," and anything that seemed to demand musical ability was threatening to her.

But desperation ultimately won out over skepticism, and Anita agreed at least to experiment with playing the bowl and chanting while I led her through a guided visualization. Within seconds of beginning the process, Anita's self-consciousness fell away. As she became more attuned to the vibrations of the bowl, her voice grew clearer and stronger, and her face took on an expression of peacefulness that I hadn't seen before. After five or six sessions, during which she grew comfortable enough with the chanting to create her own life song, Anita realized that her shoulder pain absolutely disappeared whenever she played the bowl. Often she remained free of pain for hours afterward.

Anita noticed other changes in her life—a much improved relationship with her boss, a reconciliation with her older sister to whom she hadn't spoken in over a year—unexpected benefits that prompted her to buy her own bowl so she could continue the practice at home. She has continued listening to the rich tones produced by the bowl every morning before she goes to work. Pain is no longer the all-consuming issue it once was; the quality of Anita's day-to-day existence has improved beyond her highest expectations, because, she feels, she is finally living an authentic life.

## The Technologies of Sound Healing

Using a singing bowl is but one example of the way in which sound can stimulate healing. In *Sounds of Healing*, I describe how chanting; listening to music; playing bells, hand cymbals, wind gongs, drums, whistles, etc.; and toning (vocalizing vowel sounds to change the vibrations of the body) can positively affect our minds as well as our physiology. All of these modalities are united by certain underlying principles, the most important of which is the tendency toward harmony in nature, which researchers have confirmed is indeed a universal rule.

Consider the example of two metronomes in the same room beating at different rhythms. Eventually, of their own accord, they will begin to beat in synchrony with each other. Pir Vilayat Khan poetically defined this phenomenon, known as entrainment, when he wrote about how the voice can bring us into harmony with the universe: "If the sound generated by the vocal cords into the vibratory network of the universe has the faculty of tuning one, it is because it links one with the cosmic symphony."

———

I had previously come to understand illness as a manifestation of disharmony within the body, an imbalance in the cells or in a given organ, such as the heart or lungs. Thus, the bowls, with their distinctive resonant tones, not only permitted me access to the "cosmic symphony," but also a means by which harmony could be restored within the body on the physiologic as well as the psychospiritual level.

Research exists to support my personal and clinical experience that chanting can synchronize the brain waves to achieve profound states of relaxation. Many healers, myself among them, believe that healing can be achieved by restoring the normal vibratory frequency of the disharmonious—and therefore diseased—part of the body. If we accept that sound is vibration, and we know that vibration touches every part of our physical being, then we understand that sound is "heard" not only through our ears but through every cell in our body. The sound of our voices, entrained with the sound of the singing bowl, permeates our entire being. Our pulse rate slows and our breath is restored to its normal rhythm. We enter a state of consciousness that allows us to witness our lives from a calmer, more meditative perspective.

The scientist in me wanted a better understanding of how and why this works. I therefore delved into research regarding the energetic and physiologic changes caused by sound interventions on cells, tissues, and organs of the body. Among the cutting-edge findings were the following:

- According to Dr. David Simon, Medical Director of Neurological Services at Sharp Cabrillo Hospital in San Diego, California, and Medical Director of the Chopra Center for Well-Being, healing chants and music have measurable physiologic effects. Simon points out that chants are chemically metabolized into endogenous opiates that are both internal painkillers as well as healing agents in the body.

- Mark Rider, Ph.D., a research psychologist affiliated with Southern Methodist University, has conducted the largest series of studies to date on the powerful positive influence of music, often combined with imagery, on the protective cells of the immune system, which fight invading pathogens and perform the task of regenerating injured tissues.

- Dr. Jeffrey Thompson, who teaches at the California Institute for Human Science and directs his own Center for Neuro-Acoustic Research, has undertaken pioneering studies of the physical effects of the singing bowls and other sound frequencies. Thompson has even shown that the singing bowls produce a sound comparable in frequency and tone to the sounds produced by the rings of Uranus—emanations measured with state-of-the-art instruments by NASA scientists. Thompson has translated his research into powerful treatments for learning disabilities and a wide range of physical disorders.

- Helen Bonny, a music therapist and research fellow at the Maryland Psychiatric Institute, created a process she called Guided Imagery and Music, which assists patients to enter into a state of deep relaxation wherein they articulate their sensations, thoughts, and feelings.

These findings, along with others I will discuss in the chapters that follow, have supported my efforts to apply sound in the clinical realm. Working with patients, I have developed specific approaches to healing and wellness that make use of the principles of resonance and entrainment. These techniques, which represent a synthesis of the best work being carried out in the field of mind-body, include:

- **Life Songs**—Each person's life song is a unique, mantra-like string of one-syllable, rhythmic sounds, personally composed by that individual, which resonates with his or her essence. Chanting your life song during the ESSENCE Sound Meditation allows negative thoughts to gently clear away, creating space for more productive, harmonious thoughts and feelings.

- **ESSENCE Sound Meditation**—A meditation process that uses the voice and the singing bowl or another sound source, to create a level of awareness beyond the commonplace worries and concerns of the mind in order to awaken the spirit for self-healing.

- **Energetic Re-creation**—A process that expands upon the ESSENCE Sound Meditation by allowing us to give voice to both the positive and negative sides of our emotional conflicts and inner dualities, so that we ultimately learn how to create blends of sound that help us to transcend these polarities. The result is a deeper state of resolution that furthers our capacity to live within our essence.

Finding your life song will allow you to explore your essence and discover your own innate healing abilities. The regular practice of the ESSENCE Sound Meditation will enable you to harness the power of your truest self, while Energetic Re-creation furthers this process by transforming the disharmony of polarity and conflict into the harmony of inner wisdom. The key to all three of these exercises is the sound and tone of your own voice. Singing bowls, perhaps the simplest of instruments, are the most useful tool I have found for teaching people to work with their breath, sound, tones, and resonance; I encourage you, however, to experiment with any instrument or sound method that feels most comfortable. In *Sounds of Healing,* you will combine these three fundamental techniques with the singing bowls or the instrument of your choice, as well as with the music that stirs your soul, to comprise a comprehensive approach to the use of sound for healing and wellness.

My hope and belief is that we can all find the rhythms and harmonics of our celestial music, and that our efforts will indeed enable us to live extraordinary lives—our own, authentic lives—filled with peace, passion, health, and a sense of unity with the universe.

# PART I

# THE COSMIC SYMPHONY AND HOW IT HEALS

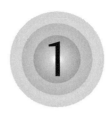

# An Overview of Sound and Healing

M argaret walked into my office, her face pale and drawn with anxiety. She had just turned thirty. A week after celebrating her birthday, she had been diagnosed with breast cancer and had to undergo a mastectomy. Her surgeon had referred her to me to map out a course of chemotherapy, because her biopsy revealed that two of the lymph nodes under her arm were positive for cancer. I saw the fear in her eyes as I greeted her and introduced myself. "I'm too young to have to deal with this," she said mournfully within moments of sitting down across from me.

As I always do, I began with a discussion of her upcoming chemo regimen, after which I answered her many questions: which drugs I would recommend, what dosage, how many weeks of treatment, what other strategies I had in mind. But she was simply too distressed to make any decisions about the course she needed to pursue. Margaret made no secret of the fact that she felt despondent and angry. She knew all the potential side effects of chemotherapy—hair loss, nausea, vomiting, and fatigue. "I'm so scared and depressed," she told me. She was convinced that no matter what she did to fight the cancer, she would lose the battle and die.

It seemed clear to me that the anguish she was experiencing was neither new nor related exclusively to the breast cancer. "Was there any other time in your life that you felt this frightened?" I asked her.

She stared at me quizzically. I was a medical oncologist, not a psychiatrist. Why was I probing into the realm of her emotions when I was supposed to be talking medicine with her? But she was obviously intrigued by my question, and after some hesitation, she recalled feeling a similar sense of abject terror when her mother suffered a nervous breakdown after the death of her father when Margaret was nine. Her mother had never fully recovered from the breakdown, and now, although Margaret longed for her mother's love and support during her current crisis, she was afraid to reach out for her help. Margaret was convinced that she'd once again be disappointed by her mother's lack of response, as she so often had been during her childhood.

When I reached over to the bookshelf to grab a ten-inch quartz crystal bowl—similar to Tibetan singing bowls, but easier to work with because quartz vibrates less than metal—Margaret moved from being curious to frankly startled. I told her that if she was willing, I'd like to spend a few minutes playing the bowl with her. At the same time, I would guide her through a brief meditation during which I would ask her to give voice to the sound of the hurt that she had carried since her father's death and her mother's emotional collapse.

Perhaps Margaret was persuaded by the fact that I had been highly recommended by her surgeon. Or perhaps it was a measure of her despair and anguish that she allowed herself to agree to my seemingly strange request. Whatever the source of her motivation, she followed my lead.

I placed the opaque white bowl on my desk and gently tapped its rim with a felt-tipped wooden mallet. The resulting waves of pure vibration filled the space between us, resonating through both our bodies. At my suggestion, Margaret closed her eyes, as I did mine. Then I guided her through the *bija* mantras, which I had chosen for their simplicity of sound and universal appeal.

After about five minutes of chanting the mantras, I put down the mallet and opened my eyes. Margaret's entire manner and appearance had undergone a profound change. She was smiling now and no longer slumped defeatedly in her chair. The tension in her jaw had vanished, and she was noticeably calmer. After a few seconds of silence, I asked if she was now ready to make decisions about her cancer treatment. She nodded and leaned forward, indicating by her body language that she was more emotionally prepared to wage—and win—her battle against cancer.

Over the course of the next several weeks, Margaret and I continued working with the bowls, along with a variety of sound and meditation exercises of increasing depth and complexity. Within a brief span of time, Margaret's experience of cancer therapy shifted from one of abject fear to one of peaceful acceptance that reflected the gradual resolution of her past hurts and current states of helplessness and fear. Margaret finally seemed able to accept that if she could not turn to her mother, she could still find the necessary resources within herself. Through this evolution, she was able to handle the stresses of cancer therapy with equanimity and a genuine sense of optimism.

Margaret's story is not unique in my practice. Indeed, it has become far more the norm than the exception among my patients. I am not, however, a miracle worker. I am a medical oncologist, highly trained in the culture of mainstream medicine, who has chosen to use the medium of sound as an integral part of my approach to healing and wellness.

The only time sound was ever mentioned in my medical training was in the context of ultrasound, the use of technologic probes that emit sound waves to diagnose disease in various organs and body parts. The notion that sound could be used as a healing modality—through bowls, instruments, or voices—was as far from my medical training as the application of magic potions. Yet I have been using sound—most often, the sound produced by quartz crystal bowls—in my medical practice for the last six years. It has changed the way my patients and I view ourselves and the healing process. I don't consider the work I do with sound, meditation, and imagery as a complement to oncology; in fact, just the opposite. My healing work has become as important as my work as an oncologist. I have come to see myself as a healer who happens to be a doctor, rather than as a doctor who dabbles on the side in what too many people still dismiss as "alternative" medicine.

It would not be an exaggeration to say that the synergistic effect of the singing bowls and voice tones when used in combination with meditation and guided imagery has revolutionized my practice. Indeed, I believe that sound, the most underutilized and least appreciated mind-body tool, should become a part of every healer's medical bag, whether a conventional allopathic physician or a traditional healer from a far-flung culture. We are so oriented to visual stimuli in our culture that we often neglect to credit the impact of auditory stimuli. That may be one reason sound has been the most neglected of all the various healing tools. But I am convinced that the use of healing with sound will soon become standard practice for many physicians and health-care professionals.

Even before birth, we are immersed in sound. As early as three weeks, a human embryo starts to develop the structure that will ultimately evolve into its ears. We become so accustomed in utero to the sound of our mother's heartbeat that infants who are exposed to a recording of a 72 beats per minute heart rate will become calm and soothed, whereas infants who are subjected to a recording of heart sounds at 120 beats per minute become unsettled and visibly distressed. Other studies have shown that women who live near airports during pregnancy will give birth to smaller babies than those in the control group. Still others report that infants will recognize and respond to their mothers' voices within seventy-two hours after delivery.

The primacy of sound is but one clue to its healing properties. I believe that sound can play a role in virtually any medical disorder, since it redresses imbalances on every level of physiologic functioning. In my experience, sound is every bit as powerful a tool for relaxation and mind-body healing as guided imagery has proven to be over the last twenty years. Moreover, it's my belief that sound works on the physical level because it so deeply touches and transforms us on the emotional and spiritual planes.

Most of us have experienced moments of deep feeling, whether it be exhilaration or sorrow, while hearing a piece of classical music to which we particularly respond. We may find ourselves weeping with joy or sadness, undergoing a catharsis that leaves us feeling cleansed, if only temporarily, of troubling and burdensome emotions. We shouldn't then be surprised to learn that sound in its purest form can promote healing at the very deepest levels of being. I am far from the first to suggest the healing potential of sound; this is an ancient concept that has recently been rediscovered. Indeed, the sacred and medicinal uses of sound can be traced back at least to the third millennium B.C.E.

## PYTHAGORAS: GODFATHER OF SOUND MEDICINE

The intellectual and spiritual godfather of sound medicine was Pythagoras, the Greek philosopher and mathematician who lived from about 580 to 500 B.C.E. Pythagoras is credited as the first person to take an organized approach to using music as a healing technique. One story has it that Pythagoras began his analytical consideration of music while listening to several blacksmiths at work. He noticed that some sequences of hammer blow sounds were more pleasing to the ear than others, which inspired him over time to create the musical scales. He also noticed that some simultaneous hammer blows sounded well together, while others produced a jarring noise, which inspired him to develop altogether new theories of harmony based on experiments he conducted on the strings of his lyre. While the historical accuracy of this story may be questionable, we know with greater certainty that Pythagoras was the first person to use music for physical and emotional healing. Iamblichus, a fourth-century philosopher who wrote extensive treatises on Pythagorean theories, noted that:

> Pythagoras considered that music contributed greatly to health if used in the right way. . . . He called his method musical medicine. In the spring he . . . would sit in the middle of his disciples who were able to sing melodies and play his lyre. . . . His followers would sing in unison certain chants or paeans . . . by which they appeared to be delighted and became melodious and rhythmical. At other times, his disciples also employed music as medicine, with certain melodies composed to cure the passions of the psyche, as well as ones for despondency and mental anguish. In addition to these medical aids there were other melodies for anger and aggression and for all psychic disturbances.

Pythagoras also spoke of how sound functions in relationship to the universe. "Each celestial body," he said, "in fact each and every atom, produces a particular sound on account of its movement, its rhythm or vibration. All these sounds and vibrations form a universal harmony in which each element, while having its own function and character, contributes to the whole."

This great visionary of sound medicine grasped the spiritual dimensions of sound when he famously spoke of "the music of the spheres." Today, we have no idea what his music sounded like, although I suspect that it wasn't highly cerebral or complex in the manner of a Bach or a Mozart. Most likely, it was "primitive," with simple and repetitive patterns, yet these types of elemental music have survived in many world cultures as healing modalities.

## SOUND ACROSS CULTURES AND WISDOM TRADITIONS

Ever since I first became interested in sound and healing through Ödsal, the Tibetan monk who introduced me to the singing bowls, I've been eager to learn more about the earliest uses of sound and music. I was fascinated to discover that sound is a universal motif in every great spiritual and mystical belief system. Consider the obvious reality that in every religion and wisdom tradition, whether Eastern or Western, many more prayers are sung than spoken. Although the spoken word carries its own rhythms and vibrations, and it, too, is essential to prayer and spiritual practice, the vast repertoire of sacred songs and chants underscores the fact that the great religions have always used sound and music to intensify our communion with the divine power, however we define or name that power.

You might wonder how the use of sound and song in spiritual myths and practices relates to physical health and healing. I have begun to accept that spiritual awakening is a phenomenon of mind and body with real consequences for physical well-being. Jeffrey Levin, social epidemiologist at the Eastern Virginia School of Medicine, has uncovered over 250 published empirical studies that demonstrate the largely beneficial health effects of religious or spiritual practice. Levin's findings, along with a body of recent evidence about spirituality, prayer, and healing, much of which has been catalogued by physician Larry Dossey, proves that spirituality belongs in the mind-body health equation. Thus, the spiritual uses of sound are certainly relevant to "sound medicine," and in some cases, such as shamanistic ritual practices, sound is explicitly used both for spiritual awakening as well as physical healing.

## CREATION MYTHS

Our ancestors intuitively embraced sound as the very essence of the life force and wove it into the fabric of their creation myths. In every culture, in every corner of the globe, the ancients told stories of sound and song and the spoken word to explain how humankind was delivered into existence. According to the biblical narrative, "God said, Let us make man in our image ..." (Gen. 1:26). The will of the divine was manifested through the power of that simple declarative statement, and the universe was transformed by the creation.

According to Hindu tradition, creation begins with the spoken word. The Vedic texts depict Prajapati, the creator of all beings, as he is hatched from the cosmic egg and utters the words that created the sky, the heavens, and the earth: "Bhuh, Bhuvah, Svar." The creator speaks, and sound is the beginning of creation.

The "Popul Vuh," the majestic Mayan language poem that recalls the creation myths of the Mayan people, describes the arrival of men on earth through the power of word: "They were not born of woman, nor were they begotten by the Creator, nor by the Forefathers. Only by a miracle, by means of incantation were they created and made by the Creator."

Many North American native tribes share this idea of sound and song as the wellspring of creation. The Athabascan tribe of western Canada believes that the god Asintmah wove songs into the "Great Blanket of Earth," and thereby created the world. According to the Hopis, Spider-Woman created all forms of life on earth, including human beings, and breathed life into them by singing a Creation Song. In Navajo mythology, "It is the wind that gives them [First Man and First Woman] life. . . . In the skin of our fingers we see the trail of the wind. . . . It shows us where the wind blew when our ancestors were created." And what is wind if not a form of breath, the herald of sound? For Native Americans, music is the "breath-of-life," and it is an intrinsic part of their spiritual practice, a direct link with the mystical forces inherent in nature.

The concept of song goes far beyond musical content for the Aborigines, the indigenous people of Australia whose creation stories date back almost 150,000 years. Song lies at the very heart of the aboriginal creation myth. Bruce Chatwin, in his splendid book *The Songlines,* described how the Aborigines conceived of song as "both a map and a direction-finder," a guide by which they journeyed great distances through their geographic as well as metaphysic landscapes:

> Each totemic ancestor, while traveling through the country, was thought to have scattered a trail of words and musical notes along the line of his footprints. . . . [t]hese Dreaming-tracks lay over the land as "ways" of communication between the most far-flung tribes. [They] . . . wandered over the continent in the Dreamtime singing out the name of everything that crossed their path—birds, animals, plants, rocks, water holes—and so sang the world into existence.

## THE HINDU TRADITION:
## OCEANS OF VIBRATION

The sages of all the great faiths used sound and song in their communion with the infinite creative force—whether that force lies within (our own essence) or without (the Divine entity or being). The Hindu tradition traces its origins to the *Rig-Veda,* a collection of over one thousand hymns written in Sanskrit during the third millennium B.C.E. A core precept of this tradition holds that song is a sacred prescription, a means to calm the mind and senses in order to achieve a deeper spiritual awareness. From earliest times, Vedic philosophers and Hindu holy men used chants and simple, one-syllable sounds (which we know as mantras) to reach a state of consciousness conducive to communion with the divine essence of the universe. The Vedic seers believed that the power of the mantras was such that their regular and prolonged invocation could lead to a profound knowledge and understanding of the ultimate Truth.

Many of the Vedic mantras are still invoked today by millions of Hindus as well as non-Hindu practitioners of yoga. In fact, an entire school of yogic philosophy and practice known as Mantra-Yoga is based on the idea that sound exists at several levels of consciousness. Those who adhere to Mantra-Yoga believe that auditory experience falls across a spectrum of awareness, from sound that is audible in our regular, daily existence, to auditory sensation that manifests itself only when we enter into a state of deep meditation.

The ancient Indian holy men understood what modern science has since proven: that the entire cosmos is "an ocean of vibration," the source of all manifestation. The world that we perceive, as well as the realm of the Divine or Absolute that lies beyond our normal state of perception, is filled with and distinguished by waves of sonic vibration. Practitioners of Mantra-Yoga use these sonic vibrations to fathom the mysteries of the universe—and thus arrive at a level of consciousness that is at one with the undivided self.

The most basic and most easily remembered mantras are the *bija* or seed mantras, so called because they are the seed sounds by which we can move into our higher consciousness or essence. The sound of OM, the most sacred of the seeds mantras, is still used to this day by many people who meditate regardless of their religious affiliation. I often suggest to my patients that they begin their meditations by chanting *OM,* which is said to contain all of life's pulsations. Thus when we speak the mantra, we connect with the stream of infinite vibrations of which our universe is comprised.

"The essence of word and sound is *OM,"* we are told by the Upanishads, one of the most venerated of the Vedic texts. *OM* is described elsewhere in the Buddhist scriptures as "the most powerful one. Its power alone can bring enlightenment."

## RITUALS OF SOUND

Whether we invoke *OM* or chant simple songs—of joy, anger, or sadness—we celebrate the link forged through generations of humankind, a link that connects us to our earliest ancestors. Singing is a form of communication that predates speech, according to the renowned violinist and conductor Yehudi Menuhin, who says that the proof can be found in the human bone structure: "Our vocal mechanism is complex—for chanting, the lungs and vocal cords are enough; when we speak, the mouth and tongue are drawn into play. Early human skeletal remains reveal signs that the use of the voice to produce speech goes back some eight thousand years while also suggesting that chanting began perhaps a half a million years earlier."

We only need to spend a short time with an infant to recognize that we express ourselves with song long before we ever learn to speak. No matter what the native language of their parents, infants the world over utter similar sounds—mmmm, mem, mum, mu, me—as they grope their way toward speech. The ritualistic elements of song traverse physical and cultural boundaries, demonstrating by example, a few of which I've provided below, Yehudi Menuhin's assertion that song predates speech.

- Eskimos of eastern Greenland settle their arguments with drums and a song, which they use to discharge their rage toward their enemy.

- The tribeswomen of New Guinea keen songs of grief to mourn the passing of their loved ones.

- In ancient Greece, Rome, and Egypt, the priests in the temples sang as they healed the afflicted.

- The story is told on the Aleutian Islands of the young girl whose singing restored a dead man to life.

- The Apaches mark the life passages of women, from young girlhood to motherhood, by singing songs.

- Women in Finland sing to the "Pain Spirit" to lessen the pain while they are in labor.

- Among the Pueblos of New Mexico, part of the childbirth ritual requires that the woman who delivers the baby greets the infant with a song.

- In East Africa, songs play a paramount role in the ceremonial naming of a child.

As I read about the transcultural use of song to mark life cycle events, I thought about the men and women who come to me each day for treatment of cancer and other ailments. What so many of my patients have in common is not the specifics of their disease, but rather their inability to hear their personal life song. It's as if the negative messages they've received and the traumas they've experienced since childhood have caused them to become tone-deaf to the true and unencumbered voice of their own souls. Odd as it may seem, many of us unconsciously prefer to ignore the summons of our innermost essence. We refuse to emotionally acknowledge our illness and find it difficult to accept healing.

Ronnie was a thirty-eight-year-old businessman who came to see me for a precancerous condition known as Barrett's esophagus, which most often presents itself as frequent indigestion. Ronnie had noticed that his disease usually flared up when he felt irritated with his two children or with his employees, whom he characterized as "incompetent idiots."

"I own a manufacturing company. If the work doesn't get done and I lose clients, I'll be out of business," he announced, glaring at me as if I were another of the incompetent idiots with whom he had to contend. "If I lose my business, I can't pay my bills. My wife and kids have expensive tastes. They would leave me for sure."

I was sure that the chronic stress of worrying that he was about to go bankrupt and lose his family were contributing factors to Ronnie's illness. I wanted him to try and examine the beliefs that lay at the core of his conflict, so I urged him to explore the feelings he associated with what he'd just told me.

He shook his head. "No, thanks, Doc. I came in for an endoscopy, to make sure the Barrett's wasn't getting any worse. No point in taking up your time or mine talking about a situation that can't be changed."

I was concerned for Ronnie after he left my office that day, because I'm convinced that physical recovery cannot occur unless we acknowledge our constricted natures and boldly strike out beyond their borders to discover our true, unencumbered selves. I was eventually able to help Ronnie make such a transition, using the methods I describe in subsequent chapters.

As children, we are programmed to survive. We learn what is required of us in order to be comfortable in our world. Most of us forget that we came into this life to experience, expand, and grow. When our lives become contracted and limited, as Ronnie's had, we unconsciously disrupt our own familiar patterns of security, creating events or states of being that we think of as adversity. We unwittingly initiate such moments of crisis as a way to trick ourselves into uncovering our essence. Such events force us to ask ourselves: Is this all my life is about? Can't I be more than my stressful job, my unhappiness with my family, my addictive behaviors, my financial troubles?

Sacred rituals that involve music, song, and dance may be useful in persuading those who are ill or unhappy to transcend their resistances. In my medical practice, I have drawn from these rituals, past and present, Western and non-Western, to develop an approach to sound and music in healing that bypasses people's psychic defenses and helps them to engage emotionally and spiritually with their illness and recovery process. One of the strongest traditions, and an influence on my own work, is that of shamanism.

## SHAMANISM, SOUND, AND THE HEALING TRADITION

Many Americans know so little about shamanism that they confuse shamanic healers with spiritual quackery. Yet shamans, who were considered mediators between the natural world and the spiritual realm, were among the very earliest people to use sound-based rituals for healing. The shamanistic belief system began 20,000 to 50,000 years ago and has been practiced all over the world, from Siberia to Africa to South America. Shamans use the steady, repetitive beating of drums and rattles to move into an altered state of consciousness that enables them and their patients to take a mental journey that will lead them back to health. My own patients use Sound Meditation and the singing bowls. Although it might seem heretical for a medical oncologist such as myself to relate in any way to shamanism, I feel that I'm involved in a similar process of embarking with them on a healing journey.

Michael Harner, one of the world's leading experts on shamanism, was himself initiated into the practice by a shaman elder of the Jivaro Indians in the Ecuadorian Andes. In his seminal book, *The Way of the Shaman,* Harner describes "the steady, monotonous beat of the drum [that] acts like a carrier wave, first to help the shaman enter the SSC [shamanic state of consciousness], and then to sustain him on his journey." In Siberia, shamans of the Tuvan tribe often use the image of a horse or canoe to characterize the drumbeat that carries them into otherworldly trance states, as exemplified by these verses from a lyrical Tuvan poem:

> *Oh, painted drum who standeth in the forward corner!*
> *My mounts—male and female maral deer . . .*
> *Fulfill my wishes*
> *Like flitting clouds, carry me*
> *Through the lands of dusk*
> *And below the leaden sky,*
> *Sweep along like wind*
> *Over the mountain peaks.*

The drumbeat that transports the shaman "through the lands of dusk" is not only a poetic metaphor; it also has physiologically transformative effects. In the early 1960s, researcher Andrew Neher studied the effects of shamanic-style drumming on the central nervous system and discovered that the steady rhythm altered activity in "many sensory and motor areas of the brain, not ordinarily affected. . . ." Neher theorized that this occurred because the many frequencies within a single drumbeat can stimulate numerous neural pathways in the brain. As well, the brain can receive a greater amount of the low-frequency stimulus normally produced by a drum because "the low frequency receptors of the ear are more resistant to damage than the delicate high-frequency receptors and can withstand higher amplitudes of sound before pain is felt."

Research conducted by Wolfgang Jilek on shamanistic dancing among the American Northwest Salish tribe corroborated Neher's hypothesis. Jilek discovered that the frequency range most commonly engaged—the theta wave range—was the one "expected to be most effective in the production of trance states."

The passage from an ordinary state of awareness to the shamanistic state of consciousness is further facilitated by "power songs" chanted by the shaman. The songs, which mostly consist of a simple melody and repetitive beat, may affect the central nervous system in much the same way that deep yogic breathing can slow the heart rate and pulse, as the practitioner moves into a trancelike state.

In a world where each member of a tribal family played an essential role, illness was a serious risk to the safety and well-being of the entire group. Both the shaman and the patient had a large stake in facilitating a healing. One of the key elements in the shamanistic ritual was the mutual trust that was necessary in order for healing to occur. The patient had to have faith in the shaman's abilities; the shaman could work with a patient only if he or she were willing to participate fully in the recovery. As the shaman entered into the altered state of consciousness to the accompaniment of the pounding rhythm of the drum, the patient, too, moved from awareness of pain, fear, and anxiety to a steadily developing sense of calm and optimism. In this respect, modern-day physicians—especially oncologists and cardiologists who work with people facing life-and-death crises—could learn a great deal from the shamanic tradition.

Yet today's Western doctors generally have as little interest in the ancient model of a healing partnership as they do in the notion of using sound, either by itself or with meditation, to create a holistic recovery process that touches mind, body, and soul. The shamans understood that music, song, and dance are inextricably linked, and all of them require varying degrees of mental and physical flexibility. I see the interplay and balance required to make music as a reflection of the harmonious interaction of the nervous, endocrine, and immune systems in a healthy body. Rudolph Steiner, the German educator and philosopher, compared physical illness to an untuned piano. Imagine, then, the sense of empowerment to be gained from using sound—whether emanations from a singing bowl, your own voice, a flute, drum, or some other musical instrument—to create a tuning device that enables you to be both the healer and the healed. Shamans have known this for centuries; we may just now be learning the lesson.

## Kabbalah: Mysticism and Sound

You may have heard mention of the Kabbalah, a Jewish mystical tradition that has recently captured the imaginations of many spiritual seekers, including such Hollywood celebrities as Madonna and Barbra Streisand. Trendiness aside, the Kabbalah is actually a rich and complex body of Jewish mystical literature that dates back to the first century C.E., and it is filled with discussions about the spiritual importance of sound. According to the Kabbalists, sound—when it is properly understood and manipulated—can enable us to soar to the highest levels of bliss.

Jewish mystics have long believed that every sound affects our bodies in a particular way. Similar to the Vedic seers and shamans, they incorporated specific hymns and chanting in their meditation and visualization practices in order to achieve a state of calm contemplation as a gateway to an altered state of consciousness. Many of the hymns reflect the larger Kabbalistic belief that the universe reverberates with heavenly song. One typical hymn beautifully expresses this philosophy:

> . . . *from the utterances which emanate from the mouth[s] of the holy ones*
> . . . *Mountains of fire and hills of flame*
> *Are [amassed] and hidden and poured out each day.*

In the Kabbalah, as in the other spiritual traditions I've described here, sound and music are intrinsically involved in the origins of the cosmos. One Kabbalistic source, the *Sefer Bahir*, or "Book of Brilliance," which dates back to approximately 1175, makes frequent mention of sound as playing an essential role in the act of creation. Edward Hoffman, a psychologist with a strong interest in spirituality and author of *The Way of Splendor: Jewish Mysticism and Modern Psychology*, describes the *Sefer Bahir* as follows:

> The anonymous author of this intriguing work declares that the mysteries of the universe were revealed to the knowledgeable through seven "voices." Each of these sonances is described as conveying an almost overpowering sense of the vast and hidden symmetries of the cosmos. In metaphorical terms, the Bahir explains, "A King stands before his servants wrapped in white robes. Even though he is far away, they can still hear his voice. This is true even though they cannot see his throat when he speaks." Though the innermost secrets of nature remain elusive, the Book of Brilliance indicates, if we understand the meaning of these ordinarily inaudible sounds, we can penetrate veil after veil of mystery.

It is the "ordinarily inaudible sounds" that are made more audible when we play our bowls, sing overtones, practice toning, or otherwise use sound or music to move beyond our limited and often anguished sense of self to the realm of infinite love, compassion, and connectedness. As the *Sefer Bahir* teaches, we can penetrate veils of mystery to find our essence, which links us to the essence of the universe. Through my own spiritual search, as well as those of my patients, I've learned that when faced with a diagnosis of cancer or some other life-threatening crisis, we yearn to hear the distant voice of the King, to receive a message from a force or deity greater than ourselves.

But the Kabbalists were not simply espousing a mystical philosophy; they also set forth detailed practices for using sound to reach higher ground. Abraham Abulafia, a peripatetic thirteenth-century Spanish Jew, was one of the most influential of the Kabbalists. Abulafia wrote twenty-six books on meditation and formulated specific sound-based techniques to bring practitioners into altered psychic states. He also created precise guidelines for chanting specific notes and pitches, and he encouraged his students to practice these sounds in combination with hatha yoga-like poses, in order to enhance their spiritual energy.

The thirteenth-century *Zohar,* or "Book of Splendor," contains many allusions to sound and its significance in the universe. According to the *Zohar,* says Hoffman,

> the universe is aflame with the song of every aspect of creation. Not only do the higher celestial creatures sing . . . ; the stars, planets, trees, and animals all voice their melodies before the supreme presence. Few of us are ever gifted enough to discern even the barest echoes of this vast harmony, the Book of Splendor emphasizes; but with inner devotion, meditation, and the performance of good deeds, we may be sufficiently fortunate to catch at least a fleeting strain sometime in our lives.

The *Zohar* also tells us that both kings David and Solomon were able to hear the song of the universe and were thus inspired to write the beautiful hymns and poems that were collected in the Old Testament Psalms and the Song of Solomon.

I find much that resonates to my own beliefs and practices in the Kabbalah, particularly in such works as *The Binding of Isaac,* written in the fifteenth century by Isaac Arama. This Kabbalistic treatise explores the question of how we as human beings relate to and affect the harmony of the cosmos. As Arama saw it, when we are emotionally and physically in tune with our own inner

nature—what I think of as our "essence"—we are likewise attuned to the vibrations of the universe. I, too, believe that we
human beings resonate with the cosmos when we use sound to
tap into our innermost selves.

## SUFISM: SOUND AS
## "FOOD FOR THE SOUL"

As my interest in spirituality has deepened in recent years, I've
been astonished by the rich and complex applications of sound
for physical and spiritual well-being as practiced by the Sufis. I've
devoured their literature and personally visited Sufi centers here
in the United States to learn more about this ancient, occult Islamic sect, which is noted for its religious tolerance and deeply
held regard for the power of sound and music. My medical colleagues might raise a skeptical eyebrow if they knew of my keen
interest in Sufi philosophy and practice, but I find no contradiction between what I am trying to accomplish in medical oncology, and what I've learned and passed along to my patients from
spiritual traditions.

My ideas about well-being, illness, and healing are close to the
Sufi view that "illness is inharmony—either physical inharmony
or mental inharmony; the one acts upon the other." East and
West find a meeting ground here. The famous Harvard physiologist Walter B. Cannon, discoverer of the "fight-or-flight" stress
response, demonstrated at the turn of the century that mind and
body are interconnected, and that disharmony in one system is
reflected in the other. As summarized by Steven Locke, M.D., in
his book *The Healer Within,* Cannon believed that "the normal experiences of life—the onset of puberty, fatigue, hard work, every-
day worry—all made a physical impression on the body. 'Indeed,'
Cannon observed, 'the whole gamut of human diseases might be
studied from this point of view.'"

Like the Kabbalists, the Sufis were deeply immersed in an examination of how sound and music affect the body and mind; one of their early meditative techniques was a timed period of sustained single-toned chanting, after which they monitored their physiologic responses to determine how their bodies had been affected. Thus, the Sufis were among the first to explore the physical basis of the mind-body connection, with a particular emphasis on sound and music.

To the Sufis, who perceive the cosmos as a vast, vibrating medium, sound is nothing less than *Ghiza-I-ruh*—food for the soul. In the words of Hazrat Inayat Khan, the founder of the Sufi order in the West, master musician, and author of the masterpiece *The Music of Life,* "not only the existence of our physical body but also that of our thoughts and feelings" are dependent upon the "the laws of vibrations." According to Inayat Khan, the entire universe is filled with abstract sound, "vibrations . . . too fine to be either audible or visible to the material ears or eyes. . . ."

It was this abstract sound, the *saut-e sarmad,* he concludes, that Muhammad, Moses, and Jesus heard at the height of their most intense communions with the Divine. We, too, can hope to access the *saut-e sarmad* through playing crystal bowls and/or chanting mantras, simple prayers, and meditation. These audible sounds, when mindfully invoked, lead us toward the abstract sound, toward an experience of ourselves that is nonphysical and infinite. How does this help us heal, physically or emotionally? The process takes us beyond the immediate experience of our physical pain and emotional suffering, and puts us in touch with a reality greater than ourselves—as apt a definition of spirituality as any I've come across.

Inayat Khan eloquently articulated this idea when he wrote:

> Those who are able to hear the *saut-e sarmad* and meditate on
> it are relieved from all worries, anxieties, sorrows, fears, and
> diseases; and the soul is freed from captivity in the senses

and in the physical body. . . . Yogis and ascetics blow *sing* (a horn) or *shanka* (a shell), which awakens in them this inner tone. Dervishes play *naj* or *algosa* (a double flute) for the same purpose. The bells and gongs in the churches and temples are meant to suggest to the thinker the same sacred sound, and thus lead him towards the inner life.

I'm convinced that when my patients use sound and meditation to achieve a sense of peace and spiritual ease through sound and meditation, they also strengthen their bodies, which enables them to handle the side effects of whatever medical treatment they're undergoing and advance the process of healing—emotional and immunological—that is as essential to their recovery as any drug or therapy I might offer them.

## HARMONIC CHANT:
## "GLOBAL SACRED MUSIC"

I recently had the pleasure of attending a concert given by David Hykes and the Harmonic Choir, the foremost Western interpreter of a unique singing style known as vocal harmonics, characterized by Hykes as "global sacred music." I'd read about the technique, which was developed in Tibet over five hundred years ago by specially trained monks of the Gyume and Gyuto Tantric Colleges. But I had no idea of its power until I attended a workshop given by Hykes. It was another transformative experience, one of those "aha!" moments similar to what I'd felt when I'd first encountered the singing bowls. I was filled with wonderment, hearing such otherworldly sounds produced not by an entire orchestra of instruments, but by a lone human voice, singing two or more notes in a seemingly impossible simultaneity. After the concert, I bought one of Hykes's tapes and stayed awake until two

A.M., listening repeatedly to his performance. The experience inspired me to explore more deeply the subject of harmonic overtones, which are still sung today by Tibetan monks living in exile in India, as well as by "throat-singers" in Tuva, in southern Siberia.

What exactly are harmonics? To begin to understand this phenomenon, imagine a violin string or piano key tuned to the note of C. Set that string or key to vibrating, and you'll readily pick out the "fundamental" tone, i.e., the one that is most easily audible to our untrained ears. However, the sound we hear is actually the fundamental or lowest tone, which in combination with a sequence of higher or "partial" tones gives a particular instrument or voice its characteristic timbre. Harmonics, or overtones, are the terms used to refer to the partial tones that most of us are unaware of, simply because we don't know to listen for them.

After the Chinese invasion of Tibet in 1950, many Tibetan monks fled to India to join the Dalai Lama at his residence-in-exile in Dharmsala. Westerners were finally able to hear for themselves the Tantric monks, the great masters of vocal harmonics, who are capable of simultaneously singing two or three pitches in a distinctive low-frequency style that resembles, more than anything, a deep-voiced growl. Dr. Huston Smith, the renowned expert on world religions and a longtime student of Tibetan culture, analyzed the monks' singular ability and the effect of vocal harmonics on listeners in this passage from his documentary film *Requiem for a Faith.*

> They discovered ways . . . of shaping their vocal cavities to resonate overtones to the point where these became audible as distinct tones in their own right. So each lama thus trained could sing chords by themselves. . . . The religious significance of this phenomenon derives from the fact that

overtones awaken numerous fields, sensed without being explicitly heard. They stand in exactly the same relationship to our hearing as the sacred stands to our ordinary mundane lives. Since the object of worship is to shift the sacred from peripheral to focal awareness, the vocal capacity to elevate overtones from subliminal to focal awareness carries symbolic power. For the object of the spiritual quest is precisely this: to experience life as replete with overtones that tell of a reality that can be sensed but not seen, sensed but not said, heard but not explicit.

Hearing David Hykes and the Harmonic Choir, I felt the stirrings within myself of just such a shift, "from peripheral to focal awareness." I decided that I wanted to learn how to overtone, so that I could begin to incorporate the technique into my meditation practice, and perhaps even with my patients. I subsequently participated in a workshop led by Hykes, and as I gradually became more proficient in the basics of the method, I realized that overtones have a multi-leveled impact on mind and body. On the sensory level, overtones represent a rich aural experience that produces strong emotional resonances. On a metaphoric and spiritual level, they affirm the presence of intangible and infinite force greater than ourselves, "the reality that can be sensed but not seen," as Houston Smith so eloquently phrased it.

## SOUND, VIBRATION, AND PHYSIOLOGY

As a doctor, I find it extremely rewarding when I prescribe a course of treatment that cures someone of his or her illness. But I'm also very gratified when I'm able to help my patients shift their emotional and spiritual perspective. One such patient was Vanessa, who came to see me after she'd been diagnosed with a tumor of the thymus gland. A working mother of two young sons, Vanessa struck me as urgently seeking not only a cure for her cancer, but also a way to heal the painful stressors in her life.

Vanessa owned her own textile design business in New York's highly competitive garment district. She was commuting from Connecticut and spending long hours at work away from her children. "I'm so burned out, and I hate what I'm doing," she blurted out when I asked her about her job. "It feels like I'm on a sinking ship." She stared at me in amazement as soon as the words were out of her mouth. Clearly she had never before admitted to herself just how unhappy she was with her career.

As we talked, I sensed in Vanessa an untapped source of strength that she could call upon in her battle against her disease. "I don't feel sorry for myself," she said in a strong, steady voice. "The cancer aside, I'm a very healthy person. But there's something in my body that doesn't belong here—and it has to leave."

Her clarity and resolve about her illness were in marked contrast to the anger and powerlessness she expressed about her business situation. She seemed, for the most part, unaware of how deeply affected she was by her dissatisfaction with her work. I sensed that she would have to make major changes in her life in order to heal; part of my responsibility as her doctor was to offer her tools she could use to make those changes. I suggested that she begin treatment with a psychotherapist who specializes in patients with serious illness. I also asked if she would be willing to spend the next few minutes listening to the vibrations of the crystal bowl and visualizing the source and shape of her fears. Although she was unfamiliar with these (or any) mind-body techniques, Vanessa readily agreed. She closed her eyes, and as the reverberations from the bowl filled my office, her breathing grew calmer, and the muscles of her face began to relax.

Using a series of simple images, I brought her to a point where she saw her fear as a ball that was stuck in her throat, threatening to choke her. As the vibrations of the bowl carried her to a more focused level of awareness, she gained a glimmer of understanding that her fear was not only about her upcoming chemotherapy treatment, but also the hard decisions she needed to make about her career.

Since our first meeting, Vanessa has developed an ongoing spiritual practice that involves visualizations, personal affirmations, and playing her own crystal bowl on an almost daily basis. She also continues to see the therapist to whom I'd referred her, so she can further explore the issues that often surface during her meditation. Two years after her diagnosis, she is cancer-free, and she has embarked on a brand-new career as an art director for Broadway plays. "I love it!" she told me the last time we spoke. "I feel like a totally different person. My previous job was my stress point. I was a healthy person, but I had a major block in my body. And then I got rid of it."

Vanessa's story is hardly unique. So many people rush from one obligation to the next, seldom stopping to consider what's important and what's missing that would make them feel more in tune with themselves and the world. They get locked into a state of disharmony with themselves and the universe, and sometimes it takes a crisis like cancer to force them to change their patterns and reorder their priorities. By her own admission, Vanessa had never been interested in what she described as "anything alternative," but it took only one exposure to a sound-induced shift in awareness for her to open her mind and heart to the possibility of detaching from the negativity in which she'd been mired. She says now, "I love experiencing the sounds of the bowl, the meditation and visualization. When I turned forty, I was in a terrible rut, and I wasn't at all happy with my life. I felt that there ought to be something more—now I know there is."

Vanessa's case is one of many that illustrates the spiritual awakenings possible through incorporating sound as a healing modality. I have repeatedly observed, both in my own experiences and in my clinical work with patients, that sound can facilitate healing, where meditation, biofeedback, and other mind-body methods, used alone, may fall short. What is the secret of sound? The previously mentioned mystical traditions, all of which use breath, vibration, rhythm, and harmony, offer clues to this fascinating puzzle. But though the spiritual believer in me has been greatly moved by the bowls, harmonics, and other forms of sound that stir the soul, my scientist's mind wants to grasp in concrete terms the effect that sound may have on cellular functions, organ systems, the blood flow, the balance of endocrine factors and immune cell products, and other bodily actions.

As I searched for information on the subject, I came upon this very intriguing law of physics: The universe is in a continuous state of vibratory motion. In the words of Fritjof Capra, author of *The Tao of Physics,* "Rhythmic patterns appear throughout the universe, from the very small to the very large. Atoms are patterns of probability waves, molecules are vibrating structures, and living organisms manifest multiple, interdependent patterns of fluctuations. Plants, animals, and human beings undergo cycles of activity and rest, and all their physiological functions oscillate in rhythms of various periodicities."

Scientists have also determined that there is a tendency in the universe toward harmony, a phenomenon known as "entrainment." The seventeenth-century Dutch scientist Christian Huygens noticed that the pendulums of two clocks, hung side by side, would begin of their own accord to swing to the same identical rhythm. The reason that entrainment occurs is that the more powerful rhythmic vibrations of one object, when projected upon a second object with a similar frequency, will cause that object to begin to vibrate in *resonance* with the first object. We human beings also react in resonance with the vibrations and fluctuations in our surroundings, so it follows that our physiological functioning may be altered by the impact of sound waves, whether produced by our own voices or by objects or instruments in our environment.

The concept of entrainment, which represents the basis for much of the next chapter, unlocks the secret of the healing effects of the Tibetan and crystal singing bowls and, more broadly, the seemingly boundless potential of sound in the healing arts and sciences.

In Vanessa's case, as with most people who experience the singular tones of the bowls, the impact goes well beyond the level of physical recovery. That afternoon in my office, Vanessa took her first steps toward spiritual and emotional healing. The path she continues to follow, which has already brought her enormous self-awareness and inner peace, has led her to more directly discover her divine essence. As she herself puts it, she has become aware of "the endless possibilities that are out there."

I believe we can do ourselves no greater service than to become mindful of the "endless possibilities" that become manifest when our life energy flows freely from our essence. Because I conceive of all illness as a form of disharmony at a physiologic, molecular, or genetic level, I believe that the goal of healing—beyond the most obvious one of ridding the body of disease—is to recreate harmony out of disharmony. But healing can also be a means of connecting with our innermost essence, so that we expand our identity beyond a limited, ego-based definition of self.

"We ourselves are rhythm," wrote Hazrat Inayat Khan. "The beating of our heart, the pulse throbbing in our wrist or head, our circulation, the working of the whole mechanisms of our body is rhythmic." As a doctor, I know this to be true. As a healer, I believe that our bodies resonate with the sounds produced by our voices, most vividly perhaps when we are in tune with the sound of the singing bowls. And as we resonate on a cellular level, we begin to heal physically, spiritually, and emotionally.

**FLOATING IN THE BEAUTY:**

# Homeostasis, Harmony, and Entrainment

From the most narrow perspective of mainstream medicine, the notion that sound has a role in healing is simply that—a notion without substance, a fanciful idea without concrete scientific underpinnings. Modern medicine has only one serious application for sound, and that is as a diagnostic tool in the form of ultrasound. Indeed, ultrasound is such a ubiquitous tool that every major medical specialty uses it for detailed explorations of organ systems that appear as mere shadows, if that, on conventional X rays. Yet the same properties of sound that enable it to penetrate the body and produce legible images of hearts, bladders, and fetuses offer hints about how vibratory waves of sound might also be used as tools of healing.

Why has medicine neglected the potentiality of sound? The reason should come as no surprise—the whole concept of sound as a healing modality is based on a view of the human organism that differs radically from the standard view of mainstream medicine. High-tech medicine, for all its stunning and sometimes miraculous achievements, has a blinkered concept of the human body-mind. Yes, molecular biology has penetrated the cell nucleus and revealed the inner workings of our cells' genetic makeup. But the onward rush toward deeper microscopic explorations of the molecular and genetic mechanisms of cellular functions has led medical scientists to become compartmentalized—perhaps too much so—in their understanding of human biology. Put differently, every aspect of health and healing has been reduced to the biochemistry of cellular actions.

But there is a different medical worldview emerging, one that is holistic rather than compartmentalized. This new medical worldview accepts that every biological action is accompanied by cellular activity governed by genes, proteins, and cell surface receptors. The key word here is *accompanied;* our biology cannot simply be reduced to genetic switches being turned off and on, because virtually every bodily action occurs simultaneously with thoughts, feelings, hormonal changes, immune system modifications, the release of neurotransmitters and neuropeptides, changes in cell receptors, fluctuations in biologic energies, and countless other transformations. Moreover, we are now learning that these changes are remarkably coordinated, that biological systems once thought to be separate are in constant communication, that genes regulate certain functions but that thoughts, feelings, and social experiences can actually alter gene expression.

This perspective goes by many names—holism, psychosomatic medicine, complementary medicine, mind-body interactions, and perhaps most tellingly, by the tongue-twister psychoneuroimmunology. (The last term implies the continuous interaction of the mind-brain, nervous system, and immune system.) But it is beginning to take hold, because the very tools high-tech scientists have used to understand molecular biology are revealing that mind-body communication occurs on the deepest levels of cellular function. Based on my reviews of this burgeoning research, I have come to believe that mind and body are not merely connected, they are unified. I also believe that understanding mind-body unity is essential to recognizing how sound—which has vibratory effects on cells and organs, emotional effects on the brain, and which taps a spiritual dimension as yet undefined—is the next frontier in holistic healing.

## MIND-BODY UNITY: THE NEW PARADIGM

The idea of mind-body unity, still considered radical by some in the healing professions, traces its origins all the way back to the fourth century B.C.E., and the Greek physician Hippocrates, who said, "Natural forces within us are the true healers of disease." Two hundred years later, Pythagoras espoused the then-commonly held belief that human beings were most successfully treated when they were perceived as complete and undivided organisms, the sum of all their complex parts. This holistic and remarkably sophisticated perception of the human ecosystem remained the norm until the mid-seventeenth century, when René Descartes articulated the philosophy now known as Cartesian dualism, which held that mind and body were two distinct entities, one having absolutely no influence on the other.

His theory held sway well into the nineteenth century, when a handful of doctors initiated a return to the mind-body point of view. Among the most notable was the French physiologist Claude Bernard, who spoke and wrote of the need for harmony among all the systems of the body. Bernard hypothesized that our inner environment, or *milieu intérieur,* as he called it, functions most efficiently when all our systems are in fine-tuned balance. In this state of harmony, our cells, organs, hormones, and other biochemical factors work together to maintain healthy defenses against disease and proper functioning of all our broader biological systems—cardiovascular, endocrine, lymphatic, and immune, though little was known at that time about immunology.

Bernard's work was further developed in the 1930s and '40s by Harvard physiologist Walter B. Cannon, who came to the conclusion that the human organism remains healthy through a self-regulating system of balance, or *homeostasis,* that stabilizes our internal environment, including our blood pressure, heart rate, body temperature, and blood sugar levels. Cannon perceived the immune system as the body's innate biochemical guard against infection and disease. As previously mentioned, he coined the phrase "fight-or-flight response" to describe how the sympathetic branch of the nervous system reacts in the face of stressful or threatening conditions. Stress, he suggested, covers a wide spectrum of life experiences, including anxiety, tiredness, and the difficult passage from childhood to adolescence. All of these conditions could affect the human body, so much so that "the whole gamut of human disease might be studied from this point of view."

Subsequent discoveries in the '70s and '80s about the actual anatomical links between the brain and the immune system gave birth to the field of psychoneuroimmunology, the area of research dedicated to finding the connections among the mind, nervous system, and the immune system. As I've noted, researchers have since developed a growing body of scientific data to support the theory that all of our various biological systems are connected in a complex, interlocking network that health writer Henry Dreher describes as "continuous exchanges [between the nervous, endocrine, and immune systems] that enable our systems to act in concert to . . . maintain the integrity of the body."

One extraordinary breakthrough in the study of PNI (as the field of psychoneuroimmunology is commonly known) was achieved by neuroscientist Candace Pert, Ph.D., in the early 1980s. Pert discovered that specific brain chemicals—usually called neuropeptides—acted as couriers between the mind and the immune system. Her new understanding of the relationship between the brain and the body showed us that no barriers exist between our thoughts and feelings, on the one hand, and our biological healing system, on the other. How specifically do these interactions take place? Pert showed that the neuropeptides, which she calls "chemicals of emotion," are like keys that lock into molecular keyholes on the surface of cells known as receptors. Thus, brain chemicals can circulate throughout the body, delivering messages to immune cells to perform particular functions, and ultimately determining how well our systems operate to keep us healthy and to heal injuries or disease. But the interactions that reveal just how intertwined mind and body are, Pert says, occur between the neuropeptides and the cell surface receptors.

"In the form of neuropeptides and their corresponding cellular receptors," Pert recently wrote, "our biological systems (the body) are literally flooded by our cognitions and emotions (the mind). Furthermore, our mind is created anew on a moment-to-moment basis by the interplay of ligands [neuropeptides and related brain chemicals] and receptors previously associated only with the body."

Candace Pert is adamant that we no longer should even speak of a mind-body connection but only of mind-body unity. She has been the strongest scientific advocate of the idea that mind and body are not simply linked by some biological bridge but are totally inseparable. The "molecules of emotion," as she calls them, travel throughout our bloodstream, hooking onto receptors on cells in every corner of the body. (Indeed, Pert has pointed out that our intestines are filled with neuropeptide receptors; hence the notion of "gut feelings" is not merely a metaphor, but an actual biological reality.)

Pert's work in this area has reinforced my own belief that we carry in our bodies every trauma, every negative idea or emotion that we choose to embrace. If you translate the idea in energetic terms, we become "out of tune" with our essence when deleterious mind states rule the body. But I am equally convinced that each of us has the innate capacity to vibrate in harmony with our essence. Indeed, my entire approach to healing is based upon the ancient Vedic understanding that "our bodies and our world are sound." By listening for the sounds of disharmony within ourselves in the form of negative feelings and emotions, we allow ourselves the possibility of transforming those emotions. As Hazrat Inayat Khan wrote, "the sound is the source of all manifestation. . . . The knower of the mystery of sound knows the mystery of the whole universe."

How can sound actually affect the constant interaction of biochemicals and cell receptors? We know that sound is a form of energy. You might think at first glance that energy has no place in Pert's vision of a mind-body network rooted in cellular functions. However, entire schools of thought are now looking at how biological energies can influence our biochemistry and our cells at a molecular level. According to Beverly Rubik, a leading expert on energy medicine, energy fields from inside and outside the body carry information that changes and perhaps even regulates cells throughout our bodies. Research by Stanford University biophysicist Jan Walleczek, among others, leads Rubik to believe that different types of energy, including electromagnetic energy, can directly affect how those cell receptors receive information. Sound waves are yet another form of energy that can conceivably influence neuropeptides and their cellular receptors. And if we recognize that our own biological healing systems are influenced by energy fields, we can begin to understand why sound and vibration are important new tools for healing.

## Take a Deep Breath:
### Preserving Homeostasis in the Body-Mind

Sound is a manifestation of breath, and breath is the most fundamental aspect of life. Breathing is much more than a mechanical reflex for oxygen exchange; it is the basis for all of our cellular functions, our energetic well-being, even our emotional health. Yet most medical students learn little or nothing about the complexities and subtleties of breathing. They are rarely taught to evaluate breathing as an index of health and healing. In their basic anatomy classes, first-year medical students certainly learn nothing about the dynamics of breath by working on corpses, their first exposure to the human body. If I were organizing a medical curriculum, I would start by teaching future doctors to learn how to breathe. As a clinician, I often learn as much about my patients by watching their breath patterns as I do by talking to them. Recently, I've come to realize that sound is both a manifestation of breath and a means to revitalize it, with far-reaching positive consequences for people's well-being and recovery.

My own introduction to the science of breath came long before I was a doctor, when I started meditating as a college student. Up until the moment that I sat down to meditate for the first time, I hadn't thought much about the subject. Breathing was simply something I did, awake or asleep, exhalation following inhalation, as automatically as the way I poured myself that first cup of coffee in the morning or turned off the lights when I got into bed at night. Then one day, I picked up a book about yoga and meditation. A whole new world of information suddenly opened up to me, and with it came a brand-new set of ideas about the breathing reflex I'd taken for granted all my life.

Yoga, I read, is a three-thousand-year-old discipline whose goal is to create a sense of harmony with the universe by integrating the mind, body, and spirit. The word *yoga* means "union," and its three-part practice of postures, breath work, and meditation is designed to take us beyond the transitory concerns and pleasures ego to a discovery and awareness of our highest self. Practitioners of yoga speak of *prana,* the universal energy life force that flows through and nourishes every cell in our body; *pranayama* is the Vedic science of controlling the breath in order to direct the prana and thereby balance both body and mind. I wasn't all that interested in doing yoga, which seemed to require that I contort my body into a series of overly complicated poses. (I've since changed my mind and now practice yoga on a regular basis.) But the more I learned about meditation, the more I was drawn to the practice and the philosophy on which it is based.

As I embarked upon my own meditation practice, I discovered that, in fact, "sitting quietly" was not so simple. My mind raced from subject to subject, my back hurt, my legs felt stiff and cramped. I tried repeating a mantra, as some books suggested, and I experimented with following my breath. Ten minutes of this process seemed like an eternity. I couldn't imagine sitting still and silent for hours on end, as I'd read that yogic and Tibetan masters were accustomed to doing. The best I could manage at first was fifteen minutes—twenty, on a good day. But in spite of my physical discomfort, and my inability to stop the frantic flow of my thoughts, afterward I did feel calmer, more focused, better prepared to face the challenges of the day ahead. (I have since studied Tibetan Dzogchen meditation with Tenzin Shyalpa Rinpoche, which has markedly assisted my practice.)

I am nothing if not determined, and I decided to continue with the practice. I was beginning to understand the effectiveness of meditation, which involves many elements—deep breathing, mindfulness, stillness, equanimity. But the power of breath is particularly important, because according to yogic beliefs, breath is the outward manifestation of prana, which creates a bridge between the mind and the body. Deep yogic breathing, therefore, not only regulates the amount of oxygen we take into our lungs, but also influences the flow of prana, as well as our emotional and mental states. I therefore had to understand the critical difference between shallow chest breathing—the result of years of conditioning, stress, trauma, and poor habits—and deep abdominal breathing, the kind taught and practiced in yogic and other meditative traditions.

In shallow breathing, the diaphragm, the sheaf of muscle separating the chest cavity from the abdominal cavity, doesn't move downward sufficiently, so that the lungs never fully expand into the abdomen. As a result, the lower portions of the lungs, which are filled with small blood vessels that carry oxygen to our cells, hardly receive oxygen. In an effort to compensate for this inadequate oxygen intake, our heart rate and blood pressure increase, as our cardiovascular systems work overtime. By contrast, in deep abdominal breathing the diaphragm moves freely and forcefully downward, allowing ample room for the bottom portion of the lungs to fill up with oxygen. The result is more than adequate oxygen exchange; we take in substantial amounts of oxygen during inhalation and expel more than enough carbon dioxide during exhalation.

Shallow breathing is also evidence that the body is in a perpetual state of "fight-or-flight"—the stress response to external danger or anxiety-provoking events. During fight-or-flight, which is a natural mind-body reaction to stress, the sympathetic nervous system goes into overdrive; our adrenal glands pump out stress hormones such as adrenaline; the musculoskeletal system goes into a taut state of preparedness; and heart rate and blood pressure become elevated.

When we're continually stressed out, our mind and body become frozen in a chronic state of fight-or-flight; we consistently react as if we're surrounded by a pack of wild animals, an evolutionary legacy of our prehistoric ancestors. The shallow breathing that results causes a particularly vicious cycle because the body reacts as if it is oxygen starved, which to a certain extent is the case. The body's response to oxygen deprivation, which is to pump out even more stress hormones, only adds to our anxiety, and the vicious cycle is exacerbated. This catapults the rest of our physiologic systems out of balance, including other hormones, neurotransmitters, neuropeptides, and the immune cells and substances they help to regulate.

Remember: We need the fight-or-flight response when we're

exposed to a real threat, whether that threat is an angry boss or the howl of a state trooper's siren. Under normal circumstances, once the danger has passed, our systems return to normal in a relatively short period of time. Our heart rate slows, our blood pressure normalizes, the musculoskeletal system relaxes, and the entire body-mind returns to a state of relative balance. But if we ceaselessly react to trivial events with high anxiety, the pounding

## Full Diaphragmatic Breathing

Find a comfortable place to lie flat on your back, whether on the bed or on a mat on the floor. Close your eyes and inhale deeply through your nose so that you feel the breath move all the way up to your collarbones. Take a deep sigh as you exhale sharply through the mouth; don't hesitate to make noise as you release the air along with the tension in your body. Place the palm of one hand on the middle of your chest, the other on the bottom of your rib cage. As you inhale through your nose, feel your abdomen and rib cage rising and expanding with air; allow the abdomen to inflate as fully as possible, as if you were blowing up a balloon. With your hands still in place, exhale fully. This time, feel your abdomen and rib cage flattening and contracting.

Take long, deep, silent breaths through the nose as you inhale and exhale. As you inhale, imagine drawing the air up past your lungs, all the way to the top of your collarbones. When you exhale, squeeze all the air out until your abdomen is flat and contracted. Allow the exhalation to be longer than the inhalation, and try to keep the breath circular, so that there is no break between the inhalations and exhalations.

Practice diaphragmatic breathing for up to five minutes at a time. When you feel comfortable with the technique, experiment with it while sitting in a cross-legged position, as a preparation for meditation.

heart, sweaty palms, high blood pressure, and clenched jaw become the norm. We get stuck in the fight-or-flight response, and our systems are thrown out of whack.

Deep breathing is a key to breaking the vicious cycle of fight-or-flight. As soon as we shift from shallow chest breathing to deep abdominal breathing, we send our bodies a signal that the danger has passed. The sympathetic nervous system, which governs the entire fight-or-flight response, with all its attendant stress hormones, is quieted. All of the physical manifestations of stress—cardiovascular, hormonal, immune, and muscular—begin to normalize.

## Alternate Nostril Breathing

Seat yourself comfortably in a straight-backed chair or cross-legged on the floor. (Use a pillow or meditation cushion to help keep your head and spine in a straight, upright position). Bring your right hand to your nose, then exhale deeply. Cover your right nostril with your thumb and inhale through your left nostril. Exhale through your left nostril, then cover your left nostril with your index finger. Now inhale through the right nostril, exhale, and switch, so that your thumb covers your right nostril. Continue this pattern for a minute or two.

Try to keep both inhalations and exhalations as silent and rhythmic as possible. Don't be discouraged if you have congestion in one or both nostrils; this is quite common, especially in the winter months. Try to prolong the exhalation so that it takes twice as long as the inhalation. Count to three in your mind as you inhale, then see if you can maintain the exhalation for a count of six.

Alternate nostril breathing is especially effective for calming the nerves. Spend a few minutes practicing the method the next time you feel jittery before you have to give an oral presentation or make a difficult telephone call, or in the middle of your workday when you feel frazzled and uncentered.

I teach my patients the basics of abdominal breathing in order to prepare them for all the sound-centered meditations and guided imagery exercises that I describe in this book. The boxed exercises on pages 60 and 61 demonstrate two simple methods to practice shifting from shallow to deep breathing.

The essence of homeostasis is returning the body to balance after an encounter with a real or perceived danger. Our nervous and cardiovascular systems must go into overdrive, but they must also return to baseline. Otherwise, we're subject to anxiety disorders, high blood pressure, chronic muscular tensions, and heart disease. The same phenomenon holds true for the immune system. When it is challenged by a foreign entity—be it a bacteria, virus, or cancer cell—it must mobilize all of its forces to destroy the invader. But it, too, must return to baseline. If the immune system doesn't regulate itself, we become subject to chronic inflammatory and autoimmune diseases, such as rheumatoid arthritis, lupus, multiple sclerosis, and even diabetes. These conditions arise from an inappropriately overactive immune system, one that begins to attack our own tissues. To further complicate the scenario of homeostasis, the immune system itself, we now realize, is responsive to stress. So balance in the immune system also depends on our ability to manage stress and handle negative emotions in a healthy, life-affirming way.

The link between breathing and good health is more than just theoretical; studies have directly associated respiratory capacity with longevity. On the negative side, the famous Framingham health study, which followed several thousand people for over two decades, found that lower respiratory capacity was directly associated with higher death rates from heart disease. Moreover, a thirteen-year-long study conducted in Australia demonstrated that respiratory capacity was a more significant factor than tobacco use, cholesterol levels, and insulin metabolism in determining people's longevity. The oxygen link extends to cancer as well; Nobel Prize winner Otto Warburg published landmark studies in the 1960s showing that cancer cells thrive in an environment starved of oxygen.

Given the role of breath in returning the body-mind to homeostasis, it is no wonder that deep breathing is the anchor for almost every meditation practice in every great spiritual tradition, as well as in secular mind-body practices. Hindus, Zen and Tibetan Buddhists, Sufis, Chinese medical practitioners, Native Americans, and enlightened Western healers and body workers all recognize the centrality of breath, both to healthy functioning and to spiritual enlightenment.

"When we study the science of breath," wrote Inayat Khan, "the first thing we notice is that breath is audible. . . ." We use breath—and therefore sound—to maintain harmony in our bodies. The human body is much more complicated than the most elaborate symphony composed by Beethoven or Mozart, but it depends just as surely on harmonious interplay among the various components in order for the "whole" to perform with vibrancy and meaning. Perhaps it is no wonder that breathing is as much the basis for playing many musical instruments, including the voice, as it is for physical health. Indeed, we can learn from the training of wind musicians who practice "obstacle breathing," a form of deep abdominal breathing that is essential for them to properly play their instruments. We, too, can open up our respiratory capacities through obstacle breathing, although I have found that toning and chanting are among the most emotionally and physically effective ways to transform our breathing patterns.

I consider disease, whether of the physical or spiritual realm, to be a form of disharmony. But through the mechanism of entrainment, we can use a variety of techniques—playing the bowls or other musical instruments with which we are familiar; toning; overtoning, or singing—to open and deepen the breath and restore our body to a state of harmony, and reunite our spirit with our essence.

Think back to the last time you sang one of your favorite songs at the top of your lungs, whether in the shower, at a concert, or standing alone at the top of a mountain. You probably sensed, perhaps without realizing it, that oxygen and energy surged throughout your entire body with far greater force and volume than usual. Isn't the experience tied ineffably to joy and exhilaration? Such memories and experiences are strong hints about the direct links among sound, vibration, breath, and emotional and spiritual well-being. These are the interconnections that music therapists and sound healers use to the advantage of their patients, prompting them to transform their breathing and their emotional states through the vehicles of voice and musical instruments.

## ENTRAINMENT: USING SOUND FOR EMOTIONAL AND ENERGETIC EQUILIBRIUM

Let's return to our definition of entrainment—the process by which the powerful rhythmic vibrations of one object are projected upon a second object with a similar frequency, thereby causing that object to vibrate in resonance with the first object. In terms of sound and healing, sound waves may entrain the human organism—causing us to vibrate in resonance with those waves—in a variety of interconnected ways. On one level, so-called sonic entrainment may alter our energetic states, leading to physiologic transformations, often very subtle. On another level, sonic entrainment can affect us emotionally, which can thus influence us on a cellular level. Numerous studies have shown the degree to which stress, pessimism, and feelings of hopelessness depress every aspect of our immune system. Through the process of entrainment, sound can transform negative, repressed emotions into a state of psychological equanimity that has direct and immediate effects on our physiology. Sonic entrainment can also restore harmony between our innermost selves—our essence—and the universe, thus reawakening our spiritual consciousness.

Sometimes sound entrainment facilitates healing on a purely physiological level; more often than not, it works on all three levels in tandem. I still recall very vividly a patient who came to see me two years ago because he'd suffered a recurrence of the esophageal cancer for which I'd treated him almost four years earlier. Paul was a successful public relations executive in his late forties, but when he entered my office, his posture, the look on his face, the way in which he expressed himself, gave him the look of a small boy who'd endured a terrible rejection. I sensed that something other than the reappearance of his cancer was responsible for the sadness and grief that seemed to shroud him like a heavy blanket.

I explained to Paul that surgery was not an option because his large tumor was wrapped around a cluster of blood vessels, and I suggested that we take a wait-and-see attitude about chemotherapy but proceed immediately with radiation. Then I switched the subject. "You seem preoccupied," I said. "What's been going on in your life since I last saw you?"

"You probably don't know that I'm adopted," Paul said. He went on to tell me that he'd had a great childhood, raised by wonderful adoptive parents who'd made him feel totally loved and accepted. Recently, however, he'd been in touch with the adoption agency that had placed him with his family, because he was hoping to meet his biological mother. After some months, the agency called to say that they'd tracked down his mother, but that she wasn't willing to see him.

Undaunted, Paul wrote the woman a letter, telling her about himself, and reiterating his desire to meet with her. The letter was returned to him unopened. Still determined to establish communication, he sent her yet another letter, this one containing only a photograph of himself. Once again, the letter was sent back, the seal still intact. "It was just after that that I began to feel sick again," he said. "That's when the cancer reappeared."

I wasn't surprised by the timing. It was obvious to me that Paul's need for healing went far deeper than his tumor. I sensed that Paul would rather die than continue to live with the anguish of knowing that the woman who'd given birth to him wanted no contact with him. There was nothing I could do to help Paul avoid that reality. But the greater problem, as I saw it, was the deep sense of anguish that was embedded in his heart and psyche. I suspected that his recovery could be influenced by whether or not he also treated the grievous injury to his soul. After outlining the nutritional regimen that I wanted him to follow, I asked if he would take a few minutes to try something rather unusual. He shrugged. "Sure, what do I have to lose?" he muttered.

I told him to close his eyes and take a few deep breaths while he listened to the sounds I would create with the crystal bowl on my desk. I also suggested that he spend a few minutes visualizing in as great detail as possible the feeling of rejection by his birth mother that had lodged itself in his body. Paul raised a skeptical eyebrow, but he followed my instructions. As I repeatedly ran the mallet around the rim of the bowl, his breathing slowed, his facial expression softened, and he sat silent, attentive to the ringing tones that filled the room.

"Tell me what the rejection feels like," I said.

In a halting voice that hardly rose above a whisper, he replied that his birth mother's utter and absolute repudiation of him felt like a fiery energy that was burning him raw. I asked him whether he could give a voice to that energy. He hesitated a moment, took a deep breath, then nodded. What came out of his mouth was a barely perceptible whimper, the sound of someone who wanted to die. His face was creased with pain as he continued to vent his suffering; it was as if the sound of the bowl was drawing his un-conscious pain to the surface. This release over time led him to a condition of greater emotional and energetic harmony. He began to see a therapist to further explore his issues about adoption. I'm certain that Paul would have struggled for years with his unacknowledged feelings of rejection had he not allowed himself to resonate to the powerful vibrations emitted by the bowl—a perfect example of entrainment.

Three years have passed since I first played the crystal bowl for Paul. He now has his own bowl, which he plays several times a week in conjunction with his meditation practice. He also scrupulously follows the nutritional program that I prescribed for him and visits his psychotherapist as well as an energy healer on a regular basis. His cancer remains stable, the tumor unchanging, and he is completely asymptomatic. The fact that Paul's esophageal tumor hasn't grown in two years can be considered, by any standard of medical oncology, an excellent result. At this point, he needs no chemotherapy treatment, and won't unless the tumor begins to progress. I believe that he has done so well because he has approached his healing from a point of view that encompasses both mind *and* body, emotion *and* spirit.

Paul's experience shows precisely how sound entrainment can foster healing on emotional as well as physiological levels. Paul and his tumor have reached a kind of detente. I'm convinced it's because his body-mind system is in superb balance thanks to the psychospiritual work he has done to maintain a state of harmonic resonance with his own essence and with the universe.

## THE SCIENCE OF ENTRAINMENT

Of course, my case histories with patients are anecdotal, albeit persuasive evidence. But there is also a wealth of scientific information about the dynamics of entrainment, evidence that supports this principle as a key to the healing potential of sound. Think back to Huygens's observation of the pendulum clocks swaying in concert. "They would hold their mutual beat, in fact, far beyond their capacity to be matched in mechanical accuracy," writes George Leonard, author of *The Silent Pulse.* "It was as if they 'wanted to keep the same time.'"

Physicists have duplicated Huygens's discovery and shown that any two oscillators of similar rhythms pulsating in close proximity will tend to pulse in harmony so that their pulsations become synchronous. We have evidence of entrainment in the animal kingdom; Brian L. Partridge, Ph.D., an expert in animal behavior, has said that, contrary to the popular misconception that large groups of birds, fish, and animals follow a predetermined leader, "in a certain sense, the entire school is the leader, each individual being part of the followers. The group thus becomes "more like a single organism than an accumulation of individuals. . . . In all probability, it is as if each member of the school knows where the others are going to move. . . . The fact that they never collide fits this hypothesis."

Indeed, *all* of creation—atoms, planetary orbits, herds of animals, every aspect of human physiology—tends toward harmony. Referring specifically to this predilection in human beings, German physiologist Gunther Hildebrandt said, "The human organism is not only constructed according to harmonic principles, but also functions within them."

Consider this extraordinary example of harmonic principles in human physiology, depicted in the movie *The Incredible Machine,* as described by Leonard:

"Two individual muscle cells from the heart are seen through a microscope. Each is pulsing with its own separate rhythm. Then they move closer together. Even before they touch, there is a sudden shift in the rhythm, and they are pulsing together, perfectly synchronized."

All the systems of our body—muscular, nervous, respiratory, and circulatory—are meant to operate according to a set rhythm. Our hearts and pulses beat a constant tattoo that constitutes a measurement of health and vitality. Our breathing is meant to be slow and rhythmic; our blood flows in rhythmic pulses based on our heartbeat. Rudolf Haase, a German musicologist who has written about how music affects the spirit and the body, describes this same phenomenon from a musician's point of view: "It has been found that the rhythmics of the human organism function utterly harmonically—that is, the frequencies of pulse, breathing, blood circulation, etc., as well as their combined activities."

## Entrainment in Human Relations: Origins of the "Click"

The same principles of harmony and entrainment that operate within the human body are also dramatically apparent when human beings communicate with each other. Most of us know people with whom we felt an immediate sense of rapport. "We clicked the instant we met," we say, describing how the relationship took hold. Perhaps we can begin to understand that "click" as our unconscious awareness that entrainment has just occurred. Women who share living spaces such as college dormitories often say that their menstrual cycles become synchronized. Some women have even reported that their cycles became aligned with those of very close friends with whom they spoke on an almost daily basis.

Other forms of entrainment during human interaction have been more rigorously observed and studied by researchers, including William Condon, a scientist at the Boston University School of Medicine. Condon discovered that entrainment actually occurs during the normal course of human dialogue by showing that the brain waves of students listening to a lecture oscillate at the same rate as those of their professors. He also demonstrated the same remarkably synchronized rate between two individuals having a conversation. Interestingly, these study subjects achieved brain wave entrainment only when they described their conversations as "good," presumably because there was some mutual understanding and pleasurable communication.

Condon filmed many conversations and analyzed them at speeds as slow as 1/48 of a second. He compared the body movements of the listener with the sounds of the speaker and found that they were completely in synchrony. "Listeners were observed to move in precise shared synchrony with the speaker's speech," said Condon. "This appears to be a form of 'entrainment,' since there is no discernable lag even at 1/48 of a second.... It also appears to be a universal characteristic of human communication.... Even total strangers display this synchronization."

Consider the speeches of an orator such as Martin Luther King, Jr. With his poetic phrases and cadences, this great preacher of our times was able to rouse his audiences. King's magic resulted from the vocal power and the utter conviction of his sermons. But as George Leonard points out, King's declamatory repetitions, which inspired rhythmic replies in word and sound from his congregants, were a true form of entrainment. The speaker and his listeners became so tuned in to one another's sounds and rhythms that the words carried meanings far beyond the textual.

Many would consider Martin Luther King a healer on a grand scale. Other healers, to more modest degrees, may also develop an energetic synchrony with the subjects of their healing endeavors. Columbia University psychologist Paul Byers has observed: "Synchronized heartbeats have been reported between psychiatrist and patient." This intriguing finding suggests that part of what promotes healing in a therapy situation is the entrainment that occurs between therapist and patient—the synchronization of their energies, the therapist's voice guiding the patient to a more relaxed and receptive state of consciousness.

Research over the past two decades has revealed the myriad

ways in which human physiology responds to sound and musical stimuli through the process of entrainment:

- When Beethoven's Fifth Symphony was played for twenty-two college students during a music appreciation class, noticeable changes were recorded in their heart rates that directly correlated with changes in the tempo of the first movement.

- Researcher Johannes Kneutgen demonstrated that babies who fell asleep to the sound of lullabies began to breathe in rhythm with the music.

- In a series of studies that examined how music affects blood pressure, pulse rate, breathing, and other aspects of the autonomic nervous system, participants' heart rates were found to respond both to the volume and the rhythm of the music. And in some cases, the heart rate or respiratory rhythm actually synchronized with the beat of the music.

## TRUST AND HEALING:
## THE SYNCHRONICITY OF DOCTOR AND PATIENT

The rhythms of our physiology attest to the fact that human beings are not so different from the other "stuff" of the universe, by virtue of the fact that we are systems of vibratory matter. Thus, when we say we feel "out of synch" or "not on the same wavelength" with somebody, what we really mean is that we're not entrained with that person. We can't find a rhythm that will allow for an easy, comfortable give-and-take. Although I'm an oncologist, not a therapist, I believe that one of the ways I can help my patients heal is by communicating with them in an open and reassuring manner. It's not enough to inform people of their statistical chances of survival, then matter-of-factly outline their course of treatment. We doctors have to create with our patients what Bernie Siegel, M.D., calls "the healing partnership." Siegel cites a study conducted by Jerome Frank, a psychiatrist at Johns Hopkins University. Frank tested ninety-eight patients scheduled to have surgery for detached retinas to determine their independence, optimism, and faith in their physicians. He found, says Siegel, "that those with a high level of trust healed faster than the others."

I'm not at all surprised by this outcome. What is trust if not a kind of resonance between two individuals? When patients come to see me, I speak to them in a way that is meant to allay their justifiable terror and clarify their confusion. I work to create an atmosphere in which a healing partnership can flourish, which is why I usually introduce my patients to the singing bowls during their first visit, so that they can entrain not only with the sound of my voice, but also with the sound of the bowl.

David had been diagnosed at age forty with cancer of the left kidney, which by then had already spread to his lungs. Happily married and the father of three, David is a successful musician who assured me during his initial consultation that aside from the obvious stress of the cancer, he had "no complaints" about his life. David's statement didn't quite ring true for me. His nails were badly bitten, and I noticed that his leg shook nervously throughout the course of our conversation. As a musician, he took a special interest in the Tibetan and crystal bowls lined up on my bookshelf and was eager to experience the sound. By the time he walked out of the office, I felt I'd forged at least the beginnings of a bond that would help him through his therapy.

Halfway through his next visit, David blurted out, "I had the strangest dream last night." Though I was running late for my next appointment, I felt it was important for him to talk about the dream, or anything else he might wish to share. When I nodded at him to continue, he said, "The dream made me remember that up until I was about ten years old, I used to wet my bed." He paused, anxiously waiting for me to comment.

"That must have been hard for you," I said quietly and went on to explain that today we know much more about bed-wetting, which usually occurs among preadolescents whose brains are slow to produce the chemical that controls bladder function during sleep.

He nodded. "My brothers used to tease me horribly about it," he said, his voice thickening with emotion. "My middle name is Eddie. They called me 'Wettie.'"

He paused again, almost as if he expected me to burst out laughing, as his brothers must have done three decades earlier. "Kids can be very cruel," I said.

In a misguided attempt to "help" David with his problem, his parents had bought a device that they placed under his bed sheet, which would activate an alarm as soon as the sheet got wet. "You can't imagine how embarrassed I was whenever that damn thing went off," David said bitterly. "I felt so helpless. The more I tried to control myself, the more I failed. Sometimes I felt like I'd rather die than hear that sound again." He looked up at me and shook his head. "I've never told anyone else about this."

I thanked David for confiding in me and told him I believed that doing so could only benefit his recovery. My sense is that the calm, inviting tone of my voice, and the sense of trust that developed during our first meeting, had allowed David to open up to me. Having been "entrained" in this way by my vocal tone and presence, he was then receptive to the soothing sound of the bowls, which he ultimately integrated into his daily life as part of his emotional and spiritual recovery. I had the distinct image that the bowl sounds had replaced in David's mind the harsh, terrifying clang of the alarm, creating a life-promoting resonance that would prove extremely helpful to him as he fought for survival. In addition to his use of "sound medicine," he underwent rigorous nutritional and other immune-enhancing therapies. Today, two years later, David remains in complete remission from his cancer, and the shame he carried from his childhood seems finally to have been given a proper burial.

## THE "HUM" OF ENTRAINMENT: BELLS, WHISTLES, AND BOWLS

The use of sonic entrainment for healing is a concept that's almost as old as the beginnings of time. In the previous chapter, I talked about shamanic healing and altered states of consciousness that were induced through rhythmic drumming. Clearly, the shamans and medicine men and women of ancient cultures used entrainment for healing purposes; more recently, scientists have identified ways in which our physiology is altered by these sound rituals. In her book *Imagery in Healing,* Jeanne Achterberg cites an analysis of shamanic drumming that showed that the rhythmic beats encompass a frequency range of .8 to 5.0 cycles per second, which she notes as having "theta driving capacity." Achterberg is referring to theta brain waves, a frequency we attain when in profound states of relaxation, states most notably achieved in waking consciousness by masters of Buddhist meditation. This research suggests that sound, here in the context of a shamanic ritual, can entrain brain waves in a manner that is clinically significant, both for altered states of consciousness and for healing. Theta states are considered a bridge between conscious and unconscious processes, rarely traveled routes to profound self-understanding and physical regeneration.

Tibetan Buddhist meditators use two small bells shaped like tiny cymbals called Ting-Sha's. In meditation rituals, the Ting-Sha's are rung together, and each produces a slightly different tone. Careful studies have shown that this tonal difference causes the bells to emit Extremely Low Frequency (ELF) sounds between

4 and 8 cycles per second. This is the range of brain waves that occurs during meditation, and the bells therefore entrain brain waves to these same frequencies. It is no wonder that Ting-Sha's have been used for centuries to initiate meditation: They signify the start of practice, and they can actually help to induce the state of profound relaxation that often accompanies meditation. Another healing instrument used by ancient Inca and Mayan cultures was a complex whistle, known usually as a Peruvian whistle, a vessel shaped like a pipe used in sets of seven to produce extraordinarily resonant sounds. Researchers Stephen Garret and Daniel Statnekov used sensitive frequency meters and spectrum analyzers to test the range of tones produced by Peruvian whistles. As reported in a 1988 article in the *New York Times,* they discovered that the whistles produced deep lower notes, low frequency sounds that could not be tape-recorded and were audible only to the human ear. "The idea is that these low frequency sounds were important religious rituals for changing states of consciousness," said Dr. Garret.

In Chapter Four, I will detail the scientific evidence that the Tibetan singing bowls I use in my clinical practice have a variety of "entraining" effects on human physiology. Suffice it to say that the bowls, in the tradition of shamanic drumming, Ting-Sha's, and Peruvian whistles, have effects on mind, brain, and body that are conducive to health and healing. In a sense, I have tried to integrate an aspect of ritual shamanic practice into my modern-day oncology practice, a marriage that might seem an odd fit. But the use of sound in rituals of healing is rooted in more than superstition; it is based, at least in part, on the foundations of sonic entrainment, a now well-documented phenomenon.

"Our ability to *have* a world depends on our ability to entrain with it," says George Leonard. Our ability to entrain or experience our harmony with the vibrations of those around us allows us to feel our connection with the world. Without entrainment—the basis of all communication—we would exist in isolation rather than in harmony with the universe. Healing then is fundamentally the restoration of harmony from disharmony, which allows us to reconnect with our own life energy or essence.

In my explorations of sound medicine, I have come to recognize the scientific and logical basis for practices that might seem "soft," or otherwise baseless. The concept of entrainment, an interface between physics and biology, helped me to realize that sound was a force with physiologic consequences. When properly mobilized, sound can specifically entrain the human organism toward the greater harmony and homeostasis that it requires to remain vibrant and to regenerate after injury or illness. Sound and breath are one, and practices of toning, chanting, and singing revitalize breath—itself a key to harmony and homeostasis. These properties of sound medicine—entrainment, harmony, and homeostasis—represent the rational *and* spiritual foundation for a new movement in the healing arts and sciences.

## 3

## THE POWER OF MUSIC AND VOICE:

# Healing Through Tone, Rhythm, and Song

As far back as biblical times, music was understood to be an instrument of healing. According to the Book of Samuel I, when King Saul was beset by "an evil spirit from the Lord," his servants counseled him to find a harpist whose playing might mend his troubled soul. A young shepherd named David, reputed to be a skilled musician, was quickly summoned; David "took a harp and played with his hand so Saul was refreshed and was well, and the evil spirit departed from him." (1 Sam. 16:23)

David's performance may be the first *recorded* instance of music as therapy. But Joseph Moreno, a music therapist and longtime student of shamanic and other ancient healing cultures, has pointed out that modern music therapy—in its very broadest definition and application—is an outgrowth of the thirty-thousand-year-old shamanic tradition of sound as healer.

The roots of music therapy as a healing profession go back to World War II, when musicians offered to play for the entertainment of wounded servicemen. They eventually started to see results that ranged far beyond the initial goal of providing a diversion from the boredom and routine of hospital life. The benefits reaped as a result of regularly scheduled performances included a lessening of depression, greater socialization among the patients, enhanced morale, increased emotional expression, and improved contact with reality. Since then, music therapy has increasingly come to be recognized as a practical and productive application for a wide range of physical, emotional, and mental conditions.

An extensive body of research now exists that has measured and validated the psychological and physiological benefits of music on human development and behavior. But we must not forget the shamanic model: Music, whether produced by voice, instrument, or the two in concert, restores our connection with our essence—the realm beyond our conscious awareness—and thus, with the cosmos. Composer Steven Halpern, Ph.D., has been a leader and researcher in the field of sound and healing since 1970. "Being in harmony with oneself and the Universe may be more than a poetic concept," says Halpern, who was among the first to use crystal bowls and guided imagery to shift brain waves into alpha and theta states, and thus achieve a state of re-laxation that he believes is highly conducive to healing.

Carl Jung, the pioneering psychoanalyst who brought spiri-tuality into psychotherapy through the exploration of myth and archetype, discovered the therapeutic merits of music thanks to an encounter with Margaret Tilly, a music therapist and concert pianist. During a 1956 visit with Tilly at his home in Switzerland, he testily informed her, "I have heard everything and all the great performers, but I never listen to music any more. It exhausts and irritates me."

Tilly was surprised by his vehemence, particularly given the presence in his "large, dark cozy living room" of "a Bechstein grand piano with its top raised." When she inquired why he had given up music, he replied, "Because music is dealing with such deep archetypal material, and those who play don't realize this."

Nevertheless, he was sufficiently curious about her profession that as soon as they'd finished their tea, he said, "I want you to treat me exactly as though I were one of your patients. . . . Let's go to the piano."

"Feeling slightly as though I were living a dream, I began to play," Tilly recalled. ". . . he was obviously moved. . . . 'I don't know what is happening to me,' he said. 'What are you doing?'

"He fired question after question at me. 'In such and such a case what would you try to accomplish? What would you do? Don't just tell me, show me.' I told him many case histories; we worked for more than two hours. . . . Finally he burst out with, 'This opens up whole new avenues of research I'd never even dreamed of, not because of what you've said, but what I have actually felt and experienced. I feel that from now on music should be an essential part of every analysis. This reaches the deep archetypal work with patients.'"

Jung's sweeping dictum has yet to be fulfilled, but the role of music in the therapeutic process continues to be increasingly accepted. For example, the groundbreaking work of Helen Bonny, Ph.D., which I discuss below, draws upon the fertile resources of classical music, imagery, dream interpretation, and Jungian mythology, to achieve notable moments of healing and growth. Thus, when I talk about music therapy, I am informed by the all-encompassing visions of Jung, Moreno, and other clinicians and researchers. One such is Cathy E. Guzzetta, Ph.D., R.N., a leader in the field of holistic nursing and a proponent of "nursing the music of the soul." Guzzetta has explored the concept of music therapy as a process that "seeks to achieve its effects by listening to vibrational sound."

"Musical vibrations," she writes, "theoretically could help restore regulatory function to a body out of tune (i.e., during times of stress and illness) and help maintain and enhance regulatory function to a body in tune. The therapeutic appeal of music may lie in its vibrational language and ability to help bring the body-mind-spirit in alignment with it own fundamental frequency without having to appeal to the left brain to work."

My belief in sound and music as instruments of healing was born of my own experiences, rather than of hard scientific evidence. But as a doctor, I like to know how and why things work, so I went searching for studies that proved what I intuitively knew to be true. I was pleased to find fascinating clinical research that corroborated the anecdotal proof I had been informally compiling.

## Music Can Change Physiology

The first category of evidence that music has healing potential involves the effects of music on a variety of physiologic functions and parameters.

- **Reduced anxiety, heart and respiratory rates:** Forty patients who had suffered recent heart attacks were exposed to "relaxing music," then assessed for heart rate, respiratory rate, and measurable states of anxiety. Results indicated statistically significant reductions in all three measures, which suggested to researchers that the use of music may be an effective way to reduce high levels of anxiety among heart patients.

- **Reduced cardiac complications:** Cathy Guzzetta reported that among patients who had been recently admitted to a coronary care unit after suffering heart attacks, those who were exposed to music for two days had fewer complications than those who were not.

- **Lowered blood pressure:** A 1989 study reported that systolic blood pressure was significantly reduced in nine subjects who listened to two albums, both of which had average beats of fewer than 55 hertz (the number of cycles per second at which a sound wave vibrates): *Essence: Crystal Meditations,* an album for piano and synthesizer composed by Don Campbell, and *Timeless Lullaby,* by Daniel Kobialka.

- **Reduced blood pressure and heart rate:** Other experiments that used recordings of varying musical styles suggest that both systolic and diastolic blood pressure may be lowered by as much as five points (mm/Hg) per listening session. Heart rate may decrease by four to five beats per minute.

- **Blood pressure and excessive noise:** Conversely, *too much noise,* which can set off the fight-or-flight response, can increase blood pressure by as much as 10 percent.

- **Reduced blood pressure, heart rate, and noise sensitivity in heart surgery patients:** Researchers examined whether listening to music could calm the nervous system and thus facilitate recovery among postsurgical cardiac patients in noisy critical care units. Forty patients, both those who were shown to be highly sensitive to noise and those who exhibited less sensitivity, were tested the day after surgery for heart rate and arterial blood pressure following fifteen-minute periods during which music was played in the unit. The conclusion of this 1997 study was that "use of a music intervention with cardiac surgery patients during the first postoperative day decreased noise annoyance, heart rate, and systolic blood pressure, regardless of the subject's noise sensitivity."

- **Increased immune cell messengers:** A 1993 report by scientists at Michigan State University disclosed that levels of interleukin-1 (an immune-cell messenger molecule that helps to regulate the activity of other immune cells) increased by 12.5 to 14 percent when subjects listened to music for fifteen-minute periods. Participants who listened to music they themselves preferred—whether Mozart, light jazz, "New Age," or impressionist such as Ravel—exhibited up to 25 percent lower levels of cortisol, a stress hormone that can depress the immune system when produced in excess. This finding led researchers to conclude that music of one's own choosing "may elicit a profound positive emotional experience that can trigger the release of hormones which can contribute to a lessening of those factors which enhance the disease process."

- **Drop in stress hormones during medical testing**: Another investigation of whether music can prevent the release of excessive cortisol during difficult diagnostic and surgical procedures was conducted by several German doctors. Three groups of patients undergoing gastroscopy, which involves the insertion of a probe through the mouth and into the stomach, were tested for levels of cortisol and ACTH. The patients who listened to music of their own choosing during the procedure showed significantly lower levels of both stress-related hormones.

- **Boost in natural opiates**: In an experiment conducted at the Addiction Research Center in Stanford, California, subjects listened to various kinds of music, including marching bands, spiritual anthems, and movie soundtracks. Half of the subjects reported feelings of euphoria while listening, leading the researchers to suspect that the joy of music is mediated by the opiate chemicals known as endorphins—the brain's natural painkillers. To test this theory, investigators injected listeners with nalaxone, which blocks opiate receptors. The listeners experienced reduced sensations of pleasure, suggesting that certain types of music can boost endorphins, which have other health benefits—including a stronger immune system.

## MUSIC IN A HOSPITAL SETTING

Both here in the United States and internationally, medical personnel increasingly have come to recognize the efficacy of using music as a form of therapy for hospitalized patients who suffer from a wide variety of ailments. Indeed, Raymond Bahr, M.D., Director of Coronary Care at St. Agnes Hospital in Baltimore, Maryland, has stated unequivocally, "Without a doubt, music therapy ranks high on the list of modern-day management of critical care patients. . . . Its relaxing properties enable patients to get well faster by allowing them to accept their condition and treatment without excessive anxiety."

Given my own experiences, along with the weight of all the clinical data I've evaluated, I was heartened to discover Bahr's forthright appraisal of the role of music therapy in the hospital—and his assertion that "half an hour of music produces the same effect as ten milligrams of Valium." I'm all in favor of implementing as wide as possible a spectrum of complementary healing modalities, for outpatient as well as in-hospital treatments. I therefore believe that it should be every hospital's mandated responsibility to offer music therapy for its proven anxiolytic (antianxiety) effects, as well as other benefits. Although many medical institutions are still resistant to integrating such programs within their already existing departments, the list of those that do now includes hospitals across the United States, as well as in Canada, England, China, and Japan.

Anesthesiologist Ralph Spintge, M.D., one of the world's leading researchers in the use of music in medicine, summarized the physiological impact of music in medical treatment:

> Physiological parameters like heart rate, arterial blood pressure, salivation, skin humidity, blood levels of stress hormones like adrenocorticotrophic hormone ACTH, pro-

lactin, human growth hormone HGH, cortisol, betaendor-
phine, show a significant decrease under anxiolytic music
compared with usual pharmacological premedication. EEG
studies demonstrated sleep induction through music in the
preoperative phase. The subjective responses of the patients
are most positive in about 97 percent of (59,000). These patients state that music is a real help to them to relax in the
preoperative situation and during surgery in regional anesthesia.

Many compelling anecdotes, as well as clinical studies, bear
out Spintge's concise evaluation of music as medicine. Arthur
Harvey, Ph.D., a music professor whose particular expertise is the
use of music in healthcare, describes one such story in an article
entitled "Music in Attitudinal Medicine," which specifically ad-
dresses the role of music in modern medicine. Harvey paid a visit
to an elderly woman who'd been hospitalized and was anxiously
waiting to have a C.A.T. scan. Hoping to allay her nervousness,
he lent her his Walkman with a tape of Baroque music. "Within
just a few minutes," he observed, "her respiration slowed, color
returned to her face and her attitude was transformed from one
of panic and fear to one of peace."

A similar perspective is provided by Linda Rodgers, C.S.W.,
whose first job as a clinical social worker at New York City's
Mount Sinai Hospital provided a framework for her longtime interest in the confluence of music and medicine. Rodgers is the
daughter of Richard Rodgers, composer of such Broadway hits as
Oklahoma! and The Sound of Music, and is herself a composer of children's music. Newly arrived at Mount Sinai in 1982, she received
permission to witness open heart surgery. "It was a stunning experience," she recalled over a decade later. "More than anything,
I was startled by the cacophony of sounds: the sharp clang of
metal instruments hitting metal pans; the banging, knocking,
clatter of other equipment and instruments being readied for the

next procedure; insistent throbbing, thumping beats of all the operating room machinery, each with its own distinct rhythmic level of auditory intensity; the piercing, ringing of the alarms, and jarring noise from other monitors; and the sound of Frank Sinatra piped in over two loudspeakers because the surgeon liked Sinatra."

Rodgers began researching the medical literature for studies on how much people remembered while under anesthesia. The data confirmed what her patients were telling her. "The auditory pathway, unlike all other sensory systems, has an extra relay. Auditory fibers are not affected by anesthetics, so they continue to transmit sound. Simply stated: *We never stop hearing!*"

Her findings motivated Rodgers to establish the Audio Prescriptives Foundation, which creates tapes that combine reassuring guided imagery with anxiolytic music, to be used before, during, and after surgery. Rodgers recently participated in a not yet published three-year study conducted at New York Hospital to determine whether music affected anxiety levels among men undergoing surgery for prostate cancer. The patients who listened to Rodgers's tape—as opposed to those who listened to music tapes of their own choosing, or no music at all—showed an increase in finger temperature, an indicator of diminished anxiety. As well, notes Rodgers, "ninety-five percent of the patients who listened to my tapes said they were delighted to have had that benefit, would listen to them again, and would recommend them to other patients."

One recent clinical trial demonstrated the remarkable effects of a guided imagery audiotape with lush musical accompaniment for patients before and during surgery. Guided imagery pioneer and psychotherapist Belleruth Naparstek developed an imagery tape for surgical patients that transports them to a place of safety, through the use of images that suggest positive surgical outcomes: the body knitting together bone and skin to speed healing, the blood delivering needed nutrients to the area. In warm, sympathetic tones, Naparstek encourages listeners to visualize supportive entities—loved ones, angels, the dearly departed—whom they might want to be with them in the O.R. The tape, which is intended to promote a sense of spiritual connectedness, is scored with specially composed music to evoke these images and to offer its own soothing effects.

The study was conducted by anesthesiologist Henry Bennett, M.D., a pioneer in the field of mind-body interventions for surgery. Bennett randomly assigned 335 surgical patients to one of five groups, four of which listened to mind-body tapes for several days before and during surgery, along with one control group that listened only to whooshing noises. Each of the four treatment groups listened to very different tapes: (1) Bennett's own instructions on imagining positive surgical outcomes; (2) simple relaxation followed by soothing music; (3) a "hemi-sync" relaxation tape that delivered different tones into each ear at different frequencies, designed to slow brain waves and induce relaxation; and (4) Naparstek's elaborate imagery-and-music tape.

Dr. Bennett was particularly interested in surgical outcomes, and when he tallied his data he was surprised by the results. Naparstek's tape was the only one that proved to have significant value in promoting the healing process after surgery. At statistically significant levels, patients who listened to her tapes lost less blood (i.e., only 200 cubic centimeters compared with 350 cubic centimeters in the control group); they also stayed in the hospital, on average, one full day less than those in the control group.

Bennett's important clinical trial suggests that the combination of custom-tailored imagery with music has a more pronounced healing effect on surgical patients than the use of imagery or music alone. In her own evaluation of the success of her tape, Naparstek gives much credit to the emotional and sensory effects of the accompanying music. But she also cites the transpersonal power of her sounds and images. "What works best is taking people beyond ordinary time into a different state of consciousness, preferably where they drop into their hearts," she explained. "The tape is putting them in a place of love and power where they feel safe."

———

The effects of music on the human nervous system is perhaps best illustrated by cases of patients with severe neurologic disorders who respond dramatically to treatment. The movie *Awakenings* told the story of renowned neurologist Oliver Sacks, M.D., and his work with patients suffering from Parkinson's disease. Sacks has been involved since the inception of the Institute for Music and Neurologic Function at Beth Abraham Health Services, in the Bronx, New York, along with director of music therapy, Connie Tomaino, D.A, Ht.-B.C. The two have collaborated to develop a far-reaching and innovative program that has achieved seemingly miraculous results with patients whose bodies had been virtually frozen for years because of the crippling effects of Parkinson's. "For people who have motor problems, music acts as a catalyst. Hearing a beat can be enough to carry a person from thinking to moving," says Tomaino. Even patients who previously couldn't walk have been able to "bound out of their chairs and start dancing as long as the music was present." Research conducted at Beth Abraham has shown that music therapy can enable Parkinson's patients to regain some level of mobility, a finding with positive implications for people who have suffered strokes and other neurological impairments.

At a 1991 Senate special committee meeting on aging that focused on the treatment of neurological ailments with music therapy, Sacks told the story of a Parkinson's patient named Rosalie who remained immobile for hours at a time, except when she was seated at the piano. "She can play the piano beautifully," Sacks testified, ". . . and when she plays her Parkinsonism disappears, and all is ease and fluency and freedom and normality."

I can't help but be moved and persuaded by the work of Sacks and Tomaino, as well as that of Ginger Clarkson, a music therapy instructor at Yale University. In an article that was published in *The Association for Music and Imagery Journal,* Clarkson reports the case of Jerry, an autistic twenty-six-year-old man who hadn't yet learned to speak when he went into treatment with her. Jerry was deemed to have a mental age between two and eight years old, and he was prone to extremely self-destructive tantrums during which he would repeatedly bang his head against the floor or wall.

Clarkson initiated the therapy by having Jerry beat on drums, dance to various forms of taped music, and play different musical instruments. She later introduced him to facilitated communication, a cutting-edge treatment technique that involves the use of a handheld computer designed to enable autistic people to verbally express their feelings. In time, Jerry was able to communicate his emotions to Clarkson in clear, vivid, and often humorous terms. (He tapped out one message to Clarkson that ended, "We dance very well together can we dance for longer periods of time.")

Jerry and a graphic designer who works with Clarkson eventually joined forces to launch a profitable greeting card company, which Jerry named "Flew the Coop"; he now writes many of the messages and helps to design the cards. Thanks in part to sound and music therapy, this previously inarticulate and barely approachable young man has evolved into a capable, communicative, and productive individual who is fulfilling his previously untapped creative potential.

## MUSIC DURING PREGNANCY
## AND CHILDBIRTH

The positive effects of music therapy before and during labor has been affirmed by a number of studies conducted over the last fifteen years. Fifty percent of women who listened to music during childbirth didn't need any anesthesia, according to research conducted at one Austin, Texas, medical center. "Music stimulation increases endorphin release and this decreases the need for medication. It also provides a distraction from pain and relieves anxiety," noted an author of the study.

A group of women in Vancouver, Canada, participated in a music therapy program intended to (1) reduce anxiety and encourage relaxation during late pregnancy; (2) offer alternatives to medication for pain management during labor; and (3) influence pre- and postnatal development. The mothers-to-be showed reduced anxiety and "a high level of satisfaction with the childbirth experience and the ability to soothe the infant through prenatal music."

A third study used periods of music alternating with periods of silence during labor to promote relaxation and provide a distraction from pain and noise. Based on recorded behavioral measures of tension and relaxation, and patient questionnaires completed after childbirth, researchers concluded that the women had lowered responses to pain during the periods when music was played.

The benefits of sound and music aren't limited to operating and labor rooms, but also extend to the neonatal units. Research conducted with infants in a Provo, Utah, intensive care unit indicated that babies who were sung or spoken to on a regular basis were released from the unit three days earlier, digested more calories, and gained more weight than a comparable group of infants that wasn't exposed to specific periods of adult speech or song.

In a Tallahassee, Florida, hospital, premature and newborn infants with low birth weight who were played hourlong tapes of lullabies and children's songs lost 50 percent less weight and spent an average of five fewer days in the hospital.

## MUSIC FOR THE DYING

Music has been shown to facilitate not just quality of life for medical patients, but also quality of death for the terminally ill. In both hospitals and hospices, specific forms of music are being used to ease the passage from a state of pain and suffering to the realm of infinite peace and ultimate healing. The word *thanatology* refers to the study of the psychological and social aspects of death and dying; Therese Schroeder-Sheker is perhaps the foremost proponent in the United States of the new/old practice of music thanatology, which she calls the "extended art of palliative medicine."

Schroeder-Sheker stumbled upon her calling while working at a home for the elderly. Distressed by the careless way in which bodies of recently deceased residents were treated, she consulted a priest, who told her simply, "Protect them." Soon after, she found herself in the room of a dying patient, "who was sometimes vicious, often brittle and selfish. . . . He could take no more in, could swallow no more. . . . The room was filled with his fear and agony." On an impulse, she closed the door, climbed into his bed, and positioned herself behind him so that she supported his weight with her "head and heart lined up behind his." Gently rocking his feeble body, she sang the "Mass of the Angels" and other liturgical chants; the man seemed to relax against her body, until she felt as if they were breathing in unison.

Schroeder-Sheker held the man until long after he died in her arms. "The silence that replaced the man's struggle and was present in his room has continued to penetrate the core of my life even twenty years later," she has written. More than a decade afterward, during which she continued her "musical deathbed vigil," she discovered that music thanatology is a time-honored ritual that dates back to medieval France and the monastery at Cluny. The Cluny monks dedicated themselves in part to commemorating the dead; they understood that their mission involved assisting those who were dying to have what Schroeder-Sheker describes as "a blessed death" through the medium of chanting and music.

Schroeder-Sheker subsequently established the Chalice of Repose Project, a hospice program headquartered since 1992 at St. Patrick Hospital in Missoula, Montana. Not only has her work been officially accepted there as a medical modality, but the project now runs a two-year, graduate-level certification program that trains students to combine harp, plainsong chanting, and singing so that they can weave "tonal substance responsorially over, around, and above the physical body of the patient . . . the *sound anointing.*"

She and her colleagues have participated in over 1,900 deathbed vigils, tending to people who were dying of cancer, AIDS, respiratory disease, progressive degenerative illnesses, and severe burn injuries. "It is the task of the Chalice worker," Schroeder-Sheker says, "to free the physical body from literal time, burdened time, to be replaced with eternity. The music helps the body and soul unbind (not destroy) the threads that sustain life processes by freeing patients from time. Perhaps it is the mirror-opposite of entrainment; perhaps it is a macrocosmic entrainment."

## MOTHERS, MOZART, AND MIRACLES:
### THE TOMATIS EFFECT

Earlier, I talked about Alfred Tomatis, M.D., the French physician who cured a community of French monks of their malaise by reinstating their daily ritual of singing Gregorian chants for many hours at a time. It is difficult to overestimate—or easily summarize—the scope of Tomatis's life work, which encompasses almost fifty years of exploring the question of how we hear as opposed to how we listen. The Tomatis Effect, his theory so-named by the French Academy of Medicine, is founded on Tomatis's thesis that "the voice can only reproduce what the ear can hear." A brilliant physician who specialized in treating the ear, nose, and throat, Tomatis undertook to examine the question of what we hear in utero, and how those sounds affect us pre- and postnatally. Researchers in the 1960s discovered that the ear is fully evolved by the time the fetus is four and a half months old; Tomatis believes that hearing starts at an even earlier stage.

"The fetus hears an entire range of predominantly low-frequency sounds," he wrote in *The Conscious Ear,* his fascinating autobiographical account of his career-long investigation of the auditory process and how it affects every aspect of our development and functioning. "The universe of sound in which the embryo is submerged is remarkably rich in sound qualities of every kind. . . . And then its mother's voice asserts itself in this context . . . a noise in the form of a coded message of exceptional quality."

But why, Tomatis wondered, are we human beings driven to communicate through sound and speech? His answer is as profound as anything I've read on the subject of the human consciousness. "By his very structure, man is a kind of receiving antenna of a self-expressive universe which reveals its true presence. Man is plunged into an apparently limitless environment, the true manifestation of an unfathomable presence which everything reveals, which everything registers as its phenomenological answer. In short . . . I prefer to say that it is only God who speaks, and man exists to translate this message—very awkwardly it is true—into human language."

His understanding of how we translate this message was based, in part, on the observations of Nobel Prize winner Konrad

Lorenz, considered the founder of the field of ethology (the scientific study of animal behavior). Lorenz reported that the ducklings born of eggs to which he had spoken waddled toward him as soon as they heard his voice.

But did "tropism," as Tomatis termed this tendency, exist among humans? Apparently so, according to an experiment conducted by his former teacher, Andre Thomas, a physician whom Tomatis considered among France's greatest neurologists. As part of his research of neonatal behavior, Thomas had a group of adults gather around an infant within the ten-day period after its birth. One after another, they spoke the child's newly given name aloud. There was no movement, no reaction from the infant until the mother pronounced the name, at which point, the child would lean over and fall toward her.

Tomatis synthesized these observations along with his own theories to develop a technique he called "Sonic Rebirth," which re-creates for the patient the journey from uterus through birth and into early childhood from the perspective of how and what we hear. Through the use of mechanically filtered recordings of the mother's voice and/or compositions by Mozart, patients experience a reawakening of early awareness that is psychologically and physically healing.

Sonic Rebirth is designed to re-create early stages of psychosocial and linguistic development from the perspective of the ear. Using sound to take clients back to intrauterine and neonatal stages of development can have dramatic effects with those, such as autistic children, who have gotten stuck at an earlier, preverbal phase. Tomatis is known for his remarkable results with such difficult cases, but he offers this qualification: "I do not treat children. I awaken them."

To bring clients through the earliest developmental periods, the Sonic Rebirth Process is centered on an electronic device invented by Tomatis called the "Electronic Ear." The device is a "simulator of high quality listening" that stimulates the muscles of the inner ear through repeated exposure to recordings of the spoken voice, Gregorian chants, and Mozart, from which all but the high-frequency sounds have been filtered. These are "charging sounds" that Tomatis believes nourish the brain, because they consist of a greater number of vibrations, and thus have a higher energy content. According to Paul Madaule, a student of Tomatis, a primary goal of the Electronic Ear is to "re-create the prenatal environment by means of sounds rich in high frequencies, to give the patient the desire and energy to use her listening to communicate. . . ."

Long before Tomatis began working with children, he had already earned an outstanding reputation for his treatment of factory workers and opera singers who had suffered hearing loss through overexposure to excessive noise; in the case of the singers, the source of noise was their own voices. Both groups also presented similar symptoms, i.e., the factory workers had developed poor speech articulation, the musicians were singing off-key. This phenomenon led Tomatis to conclude that "the voice only contains harmonics the ear is likely to hear."

Tomatis relies on several musical forms in his client-tailored Sonic Rebirth treatments. Gregorian chants, especially those from the abbey of St. Pierre de Solesmes, are used for two reasons: They have an abundance of high-frequency sounds; and the rhythms reflect our own physiological rhythms when we are in a calm, relaxed state. Still, Mozart's music remains Tomatis's most effective musical intervention. The power of Mozart raises the question of why the celebrated composer's works have been incorporated into a healing system used throughout the world to treat autism, premature infants, learning disabilities, vocal and hearing handicaps, head injuries, and related psychiatric and neurologic disorders.

Tomatis offers this answer: "Even before his birth, Mozart was saturated with music. I have no doubt that such a situation prepared his nervous system to listen and to live only in music. . . .

[M]usical expression was the true mother tongue which enabled Mozart to communicate with the entire universe."

Indeed, Don Campbell, a classically trained musician and director of the Institute for Music, Health and Education, has been so persuaded by the teachings of Tomatis regarding the universal appeal of Mozart that he has coined the phrase "the Mozart Effect" to describe the ways in which Mozart's music can increase creativity, calm tension, and help us heal. In his book of the same name, Campbell cites research conducted at the Center for Neurobiology of Learning and Memory in Irvine, California, where a team headed by Frances H. Rauscher, Ph.D., had undergraduate students listen to ten minutes of Mozart's Sonata for Two Pianos in D Major (K. 448). The students were tested before and after listening to the music for spatial IQ; they showed improved scores of eight to nine points for ten to fifteen minutes after hearing the music.

"The music of Mozart may 'warm up' the brain," said Gordon Shaw, Ph.D., a physics professor whose expertise is the structure of the brain's cortex. "We suspect that complex music facilitates certain complex neuronal patterns involved in high brain activities like math and chess."

In his book *Pourquoi Mozart?* (Why Mozart?) Tomatis offered this far less technical but much more succinct response to the question he poses in the title: "He has an effect, an impact, which others do not have. Exception among exceptions, he has a liberating, curative, I would even say, *healing* power."

## LIBERATING VOICE AND HEART: TONING AND SINGING

"Alana and her twelve-year-old daughter, Lizzy, were driving home on a Friday night," writes Joy Gardner-Gordon in her book

*The Healing Voice.* "Coming around the bend on the freeway, they saw a car about a half block ahead of them, making a dangerous U-turn in the middle of the road. The car was unable to complete the turn, and Alana crashed into it."

Both cars were totally destroyed, but Alana, her daughter, and the driver of the other car somehow avoided sustaining any life-threatening injuries. Although physically intact, Lizzy burst into tears of hysteria, so that Alana felt that her immediate task was to tamp down her own panic and try to comfort her daughter. (Gardner-Gordon commented that Alana had been "proud of her composure as she waited for the police.") When the police arrived on the scene and began to question Alana, Lizzy bolted into a nearby field, where she vented her shock with uncontrollable shrieking.

An hour later, they returned home. Lizzy had finally stopped screaming and felt fine, if somewhat shaken up. But Alana was experiencing severe pain from whiplash in her left shoulder, pain that lasted for many months, until she finally consulted Gardner-Gordon, a musician and holistic healer. Using light hypnosis, Gardner-Gordon encouraged Alana to revisit the accident in her mind, and to express through sound the terror she'd experienced in the moments after the crash—an abject fear that her daughter had been killed.

"Through screaming, Alana was finally able to express and release her emotional pain. . . . Her body had become frozen in a posture of tension since the powerful messages she had sent to her muscles and tissues was to be in a state of ready alertness. The scream was a message to her subconscious mind that the impact had, in fact, occurred, and now it was time for release."

Alana's whiplash pain diminished over the next two weeks. Gardner-Gordon surmised that her months of chronic pain would have subsided much sooner had she allowed herself to release her terror with sound within moments or hours of the accident.

Gardner-Gordon is a holistic healer who specializes in *toning*, which involves the use of pure vocal sound to resolve tension, release emotion, and spur the healing process. In my own sound/healing work, I have been profoundly influenced by toning practices, which are as old as civilization and have been revived by contemporary practitioners.

What, exactly, is toning? Laurel Elizabeth Keyes, who pioneered toning as a healing art in the early '60s, explains the technique in her book *Toning: The Creative Power of the Voice*: "Toning is an ancient method of healing . . . the idea is simply to restore people to their harmonic patterns." But the purposes and practices of toning are manifold, as is the philosophy behind this time-honored healing art. Here are a sampling of interpretations from leading proponents of toning:

- "Toning is a system of healing that utilizes vowel sounds to alter vibrations in every molecule and cell in the body." —Laeh Maggie Garfield in *Sound Medicine*

- "Tone is simply an audible sound, prolonged long enough to be identified. 'Toning' is the conscious elongation of a sound using the breath and voice."—Don Campbell in *The Roar of Silence*

- "Toning is the process of making vocal sounds for the purpose of balance. . . . Toning sounds are sounds of expression and do not have a precise meaning."—John Beaulieu in *Music and Sound in the Healing Arts*

- Toning is "the sustained vocalization of individual pitches for the purpose of resonating specific body areas to which the voice is directed."—Randall McClellan in *The Healing Forces of Music*

- "Toning is an activity that releases and allows the natural flow of energy to move through one's body."—Steven Halpern in *Tuning the Human Instrument*

- "Toning is the use of the voice to express sounds for the purpose of release and relief. . . . It is nonverbal sound, relying primarily on vowels, though it may incorporate the use of consonants to create syllables as long as they are not utilized to create coherent meaning. Sighing, moaning, and humming may also be recognized as forms of toning."— Jonathan Goldman in *Healing Sounds*

While the practices of toning vary to some extent, all involve the use of pure nonverbal sound to increase the flow of breath, balance energy flow, release emotion, resolve past trauma, and restore harmony to the body-mind system. Gardner-Gordon points out that toning facilitates deep breathing, because in order to fully release the sounds, we have to expand the belly and diaphragm, and thus inhale more fresh air. We've already seen that when we breathe more deeply, as during meditation, we slow the heart rate and calm the nervous system, thus evoking the relaxation response.

The emotional power of toning is particularly apparent in the work of experienced toning practitioners. Bracha Adrezin, a Brooklyn-based former opera singer who studied psychotherapy at the University of Vienna, uses a powerful combination of bioenergetic movement and toning as well as chanting and other verbal expressions of emotion to help clients, many of whom have been physically or sexually abused, to work through and let go of the memories of past traumas.

Throughout this book, I tell the stories of patients who've used my variants of toning to process and resolve painful memories and ongoing traumas—work that has led them to reclaim their essence and, often, to promote physical healing of their life-threatening illnesses. On page 99 are simple directions, provided by Joy Gardner-Gordon, for how to tone. Remember, it's impossible to make a mistake while toning!

---

### Toning Fundamentals

- Inhale through your nose. Release your breath through your mouth while making one long sustained sound. When you run out of breath, inhale again through your nose and exhale through your mouth, again making a long sustained sound. Repeat this procedure as often as you like.

- You can stand, sit in a cross-legged position on the floor, or sit on a chair. Be sure your spine is straight and your diaphragm and abdomen are unobstructed. If you're standing, imagine that the sound is coming up from your feet. Relax your jaw. When you make a sound, let your jaw hang open.

- Tone a vowel on the note of your choice for as long as your breath allows. Repeat several times.

- Tone the same sound on a different note.

- Tone a syllable on the same note. Repeat several times. (Example: Tone *OM, LAM,* or *HU.*)

- Tone the same syllable on a different note, and repeat.

- Find a syllable-and-note combination that you like, and tone it again and again.

---

Play with toning. Beat on the tabletop, hit a cup with a spoon, bang pots and pans together. Try toning with your bowl, a gong, bell, or a drum with a natural skin that gives off lots of reverberations. Do anything to experiment with sound, and with the freeing of your voice.

Toning can be therapeutic for a wide variety of emotions and conditions. See the adapted versions of several suggestions by Gardner-Gordon on page 100.

## Specific Toning Exercises

- *Cleansing and Releasing.* Moaning and groaning are cleansing sounds that come naturally when aches and pains are being released. High-pitched, penetrating sounds, or even fierce screaming can help break up energy blockages that may have led to emotional and physical armoring. Release the sound that you feel from within. It may be a bloodcurdling, terrifying scream that could go on for several minutes, until it may actually end in laughter. Releasing a scream that has been held in for decades can be a joyous, liberating experience.

- *Soothing and relaxing.* Through toning, you can provide a soothing environment for the release of tension. Humming can be calming to the nervous system, and may help you to breathe deeply. You may feel inspired to sing words of support and encouragement, or even to break into familiar bars of music or pop tunes. Trust the impulse; it often turns out to be surprisingly appropriate.

- *Toning for the pain in your body.* Stand with your feet about shoulder-length apart and your body relaxed. If you prefer, sit at the edge of a chair with your back straight. You can stand up and move around when the energy gets moving. Inhale through your nose and draw the breath down to your abdomen, so you can actually see your abdomen rising. Exhale through your mouth, making a low moan, or whatever comes naturally. Do this ten times.

Wherever you feel pain or tension, bring your attention there and consciously breathe into it. As you exhale, release tension from that part of your body.

Give a sound to the feeling. If the sound doesn't come spontaneously, begin by toning as low as you can and slowly raise the pitch until you find a tone that resonates with the pain. Continue making

> sounds until you feel a release, as if you've given yourself an inner massage.
>
> Repeat this process for every pain or discomfort in your body.

In 1963, Laurel Elizabeth Keyes founded the Order of Fransisters and Brothers, a lay religious order dedicated to prayer integrated with toning for the specific purpose of healing. However, Keyes believed that toning for the purpose of healing was not a matter of faith. "Anyone can use toning, just as we use electricity," she said. "There are natural channels in the energy of our body, and if we recognize and learn to flow with them, they will keep us healthy."

Keyes described the sense of exhilaration she felt when she first began to experiment with toning. It was more than "just a release of tension," she wrote. When she allowed the tones to emerge without trying to control them, she experienced a cleansing of her entire body. "I was convinced that there had to be a relationship between this natural body-voice and the mind without conflict, and with benefit to both."

A similar effect may be produced through singing. To the Sufis, singing is *prana,* the breath of life itself, the most potent of all the musical healing modalities. According to Hazrat Inayat Khan, the ancient singers would chant a single note half an hour at a time in order to investigate the effects of that note on their various energy chakras: "what life current it produced, how it opened the intuitive faculties, how it created enthusiasm, how it gave added energy, how it soothed, and how it healed. For them it was not a theory, it was an experience."

Singing allows us an opportunity to exercise our breath, and simultaneously become our own instrument of self-expression. Lisa Sokolov, a music therapist in New York City, believes that voice can be a "healing tool" for both mind and body. She says,

"The throat is a physical and symbolic bridge between the head and the heart. Therefore singing can become a way of developing a relationship between the mind and the emotions."

As children, many of us received the message—whether explicitly or implicitly—that we couldn't and shouldn't sing. The grimace on a parent's face when we burst into song, a teacher's disapproving frown when we auditioned for the school choir, a brother or sister's hurtful ridicule when we sang along to a favorite record or CD: Any of these experiences may be enough to convince even someone with a sturdy ego and positive self-esteem that he or she "can't carry a tune," "has a tin ear," "can't sing a note."

I was one of those people who believed I couldn't sing—so I didn't, until Ödsal taught me to play Tibetan bowls. Suddenly, a whole new world opened up to me, a world of sound where my old insecurities about my supposed lack of musical gifts fell away. Some months ago, I was asked to speak at a professional conference on the subject of complementary approaches to illness. I concluded my presentation to a crowd of 250 people by playing one of my bowls at the same time that I sang aloud the *bija* mantras. Apparently, few in the audience were put off by my voice or the tones I chanted, because I received a standing ovation!

I encourage each one of you to discover your own voice. Sing in the shower, sing in the car, sing along with your favorite soloist or band. Sing as you walk through a forest or meadow or hike a mountain trail. Sing in private until you stop listening to the negative tapes of other people's disapproval and hear instead the sound of your own uniquely harmonious voice. Then, if you wish, sing for an audience—whether it be of two or four or many more.

On the following pages are two exercises from *The Music Within You* by Shelley Katsh and Carol Merle-Fishman, certified music therapists, to help you develop your skill and confidence as a singer.

## Breathing into Your Voice

Lie down on the floor on your back. Place one hand on your chest, the other on your belly. Feel your hands rise and fall as your body expands and contracts naturally while you take in and release air.

In order to feel the full expansion of your body, place your hands right above your waistline at your sides, enclosing the area between your thumb and other fingers. Push in forcibly against the diaphragm muscle as your body expands. As you continue to resist, your ability to expand, maintain the expansion, and breathe fully will improve.

Try singing a tone or a familiar melody as you breathe in this position. Listen for the difference in your voice between the way you usually sound, and the way you sound now. Let your voice express whatever you are feeling in the moment.

Barbara J. Crowe, professor of music therapy at Arizona State University, makes a distinction between music therapy and sound healing. She describes the latter as "a looser amalgamation of approaches that looks at sound as a more direct curative agent than a music therapist might see it." Nevertheless, the practice of toning, humming, and other expressions of nonverbal sound may be considered part of the larger repertoire of music therapy, which most commonly involves listening and playing music to effect healing. All of these modes have been shown to be effective in releasing and recovering from emotional trauma, in calming the spirits, and in restoring flagging energies. The entire range of music therapy interventions continues to gain credence in hospital settings and elsewhere, in part because of the growing acceptance by the medical profession of the data offered by psychoneuroimmunologists to support the idea of a mind-body connection.

The extraordinary spectrum of music therapy applications includes the following: pain management for ailments as diverse

## Making Room for Your Voice

As you stand or sit, stretch your spine. Reach for the ceiling with the top of the spine, reach for the floor with the bottom. Let the crown of your head reach for the ceiling as well. It is often helpful to picture an imaginary string that goes from the ceiling through the top of your head, through your spine, and down to the floor. Imagine a hand gently pulling up the string. Release your shoulders and arms so they can swing freely. Make sure your knees are unlocked.

You will know you are aligned incorrectly if your shoulders are rounded, your chest is caved in, flat or jutting out, or if your abdomen or rear end is tightened or protruding.

Try sitting in a straight-backed chair so that you can focus on your spine. Feel the difference between your usual posture and this one. Breathe fully and gently without throwing your body out of line. As you breathe, feel the muscles in your abdomen and back expand. You may be able to feel your back push against the back of the chair.

From this position, try yawning and letting a sound emerge. Do this a few times, and feel the release. Then, while fully expanded, begin to sing a familiar tune. Try singing with *ah* or *la* at first. Listen to the quality of your voice. What does it feel like to hear yourself sing? When you feel ready, add words. Close your eyes, stay fully expanded, and release your voice.

as cancer and migraine headaches; the treatment of the mentally and physically challenged; learning disabilities and emotional issues, including schizophrenia; alcohol and substance abuse; stress reduction, in hospital delivery and operating rooms, as well as intensive care units; and as an adjunct to traditional psychotherapy.

I envision the day in the not-too-distant future when music therapists regularly visit and work with patients in all our healing institutions; when singing, toning, chanting, and other forms of music echo through the corridors of every hospital unit. I envision, as well, the day that quartz crystal singing bowls are offered as a healing option as routinely as antibiotics, surgery, and chemotherapy—a truly holistic approach that melds sound and high-tech medicine.

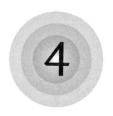

**4**

# The Healing Resonance of the Bowls

As I mentioned earlier, it was Ödsal, the Tibetan monk I treated for heart disease, who introduced me to the Tibetan singing bowls. The very first time I heard the ringing vibrations produced by the bowls, I knew I had stumbled upon one of the most potent healing tools I would ever encounter. Ödsal and I made an exchange: He taught me about the bowls, and I taught him my guided imagery meditations. Through this fortuitous sharing of healing practices from our divergent cultural and spiritual backgrounds, I began to explore a new synthesis—the sound of the bowls combined with meditation, guided imagery, and vocalization—a fusion that I have found to be greater than the sum of its parts.

Whether made of brass and created by Tibetan craftsmen, or of crystal and manufactured here in America, the singing bowls act as a medium in which our inner chaos and conflict can be reconfigured into a harmonious sense of calm centeredness that resonates through every cell of our body and mind. These remarkable vessels, as beautiful to behold as they are to hear, have become an integral and essential part of the sound-based guided imagery and meditation techniques that my patients and I use to resolve negatively charged emotions. But you don't need to be diagnosed with a life-threatening illness to nurtured by bowl-centered meditation. Anybody can benefit from the practice—and the life-affirming effects are immediately apparent.

I witnessed a graphic demonstration of just how effective the bowls can be when my brother-in-law, a diplomat in African affairs at the State Department, came to visit us in August 1998. Only three weeks earlier, the American embassies in Kenya and Tanzania had been destroyed by terrorist bombing attacks. Hundreds of lives had been lost, many more hundreds were badly injured. Keith had been working eighteen-hour days, helping to identify the dead, talking to the bereaved families, finding a replacement staff for the embassies, dealing with such immediate concerns as how to protect against future attacks, coping with his own sense of grief over the close friends he had lost.

He looked shell-shocked, almost as if he were suffering from posttraumatic stress disorder. I wasn't surprised when he said he was having trouble sleeping. Insomnia is often a symptom of depression or anxiety.

Keith had never shown more than a polite interest in my collection of bowls. I doubt that we'd spent so much as half an hour talking about why or how I used them in my meditation practice. During this visit, however, he turned to me across the breakfast table and said, "I heard you playing your bowl this morning, and it sounded so peaceful. I'm not really into meditating, but could you show me what you do?"

I took Keith into my study and had him lie down on the floor. I balanced a small Tibetan bowl on his chest, then arranged three slightly larger ones just behind his head and next to each of his shoulders. I placed two of my crystal bowls on the floor just a few inches away from him. Then I asked him to close his eyes, listen as

I played the bowls, and repeat after me as I sang a series of simple Sanskrit mantras.

I began striking the rims of the bowls, one after another, at the same time chanting the one-syllable mantras (more about these mantras later in the chapter). I could sense that he was feeling a bit apprehensive, which was understandable, given the newness of the experience for him. But after a minute or two, he started to relax. His breathing became deeper and more even, and his voice grew steadier as he followed my lead in reciting the mantras. The calming impact of the sound as it reverberated through and around him was visible in his expression, which shifted from one of fretfulness and anxiety to tranquillity and acceptance. I could see his energy changing, as well, as he started to recover from the hellish nightmare that had consumed his days and nights.

I spent about twenty minutes with Keith, playing the bowls and chanting, until the room felt as if it were filled with the vibrations we had created together. His face looked serene as I tiptoed out, leaving him alone to "bathe" in the "ocean of sound," to borrow a phrase from the Hindu philosophers. An hour later, he emerged smiling, back to his old self, and he remained upbeat and cheerful for the rest of his stay.

If just one twenty-minute session can produce such a pronounced shift in mood and emotions, imagine how our feelings and perceptions might be positively altered by regularly incorporating this practice into our routine. The stories I tell of how bowl- and sound-centered meditation has changed my patients' lives may read like a hyped-up pitch, but I believe unequivocally—and I've seen for myself the proof—that the use of sound is among the most powerful healing modalities ever embraced by twentieth-century practitioners.

## TIBETAN BOWLS:
## THE SOUNDS OF THE VOID

People have known about the power of sound for thousands of years, but few have been willing to talk about it until recent times. It's especially fitting that my first experience with the singing bowls should have occurred thanks to Ödsal, because the use of sound has been a sacred and hidden aspect of Tibetan ceremonial rites for many centuries.

A deep respect for sound as a source of enlightenment and spiritual strength is embedded in Tibetan culture; indeed, Tibetans consider the voice to be an essential element of human nature—the link between mind and body, between the spiritual and the material worlds.

Tibetan Buddhists have incorporated the use of metal bells, or Ting-sha's, in their meditation practice for thousands of years. The function of the metal bowls is less clear. As recently as thirty years ago, Tibetans often told tourists who inquired about the bowls that they were used in the temples to burn incense or to hold simple offerings of water or grain at the altars. Another common explanation was that the bowls were simply household dishes, for serving and eating food.

A Hungarian shaman, Joska Soos, understood otherwise from the Tibetan lamas he met while on retreat at their monastery in England. When Soos asked what he could do to further his spiritual development, he received the following answer:

> They [the lamas] took me to a small room and there were the bowls. I listened to them. Afterwards they presented me with some bowls. I did not have to go on a retreat. I merely had to intensify my path, immersing myself in the sounds. ... Slowly it came to me, the whole universe opened up. Amongst the lamas themselves, these bowls are only used in secret rituals by those who are acknowledged

masters in sound. They have learned to sing the ritual songs and play the ritual instruments correctly. They use the singing bowls in secret and only for themselves, not in public, and not even for other monks. It is strictly forbidden to talk about the rituals or the singing bowls themselves. This is because a knowledge of sound carries with it great power. . . . If you ask a lama with a singing bowl in his hands whether it is true that they are used for psychic, psychological and physical purposes, he will smile and reply: "Perhaps."

Recently, I spoke with the Venerable Tenzen Shyalpa Rinpoche, a Tibetan lama who divides his time between Nepal and a retreat in western Massachusetts. He recalled sitting with his monastic colleagues, playing the bowls, and chanting for fourteen hours at a time. It's thus safe to assume that the metal bowls served both ceremonial and practical functions. According to one theory, the mystery surrounding the bowls exists because they were linked to shamanistic rituals that were not an accepted part of Tibetan Buddhist practice. Long before the eighth century, when Lamaism—as Tibetan Buddhism is known—became the dominant faith of Tibet, the Bon religion flourished there, as well as throughout the rest of the Himalayas. Bon is a form of shamanism that focuses on sound and the chanting of mantras in order to influence the unseen spirits and energy forces that control the universe. (The word *Bon* comes from the verb *bon pa,* which means "to recite magical formulas.") It's entirely likely that the Tibetan holy men took great care to withhold information about their use of the bowls, because their tones and overtones carried within them a wealth of knowledge about the cosmos and all of its truths. In the words of Tibetan monk Lama Thupten Lobsang Leche, "The Bowl sound is the sound of the Void."

There are varying explanations as to who was responsible for crafting the bowls; according to one theory, they were made by the monks themselves. If that's the case, it's hard to imagine that they would have created bowls capable of producing such extraordinary sounds if they hadn't intended them to "sing." The bowls were said to have been made from seven different metals—gold, silver, mercury, copper, iron, tin, and lead—all of which were abundantly available in Tibet and Nepal. Individually, each metal has its own distinctive sound, and in combination with one or more of the other metals, creates harmonics that differ from bowl to bowl, depending on the particular alloy.

Whatever the reasons in the past for the sense of mystery about the bowls, in this era of greater communication with the people of the East and flourishing interest in sound healing, we've been able to learn much more about the bowls as instruments of healing and spiritual awakening. In my case, I've learned more about the bowls from personal, hands-on experience than from anything I've read about them.

When I played the bowls with Ödsal, I discovered for myself the power of harmonic sound with all of its glorious overtones. The sound is produced by moving a wood baton around the rim of the bowl, producing a deep, rich note with a strong vibrato. Depending on how quickly or slowly you move the baton, to a certain extent you can control the qualities of the sound. You can feel the vibrations resonating throughout your body, and when you stop, as the sound gradually dies away, you are likely to feel a lightness, a relief of pressure, in your head and body.

A friend of mine once compared this feeling of lightness to a mild marijuana high. I think he got it backward. Drugs are popular because the high they offer mimics the feelings of spiritual release that all of us crave. But the high is transitory, bogus, and can be dangerously addictive. What we feel when we play a singing bowl is the real thing: a moment out of time that offers a release from the distractions and stresses of the outside world.

Although you can still find antique bowls in stores that specialize in Tibetan crafts, the growing number of customers far exceeds the rather limited supply. No new bowls have been hand-crafted in over fifty years, and those that are mass-produced, while less expensive, do not have the same, rich vibrations as the bowls that were made prior to the Chinese invasion of Tibet. Because I wanted to recommend the bowls to my patients, I experimented with glass and ceramic versions, but the sound they produced also fell far short of the Tibetan bowls. The solution to my problem came through a chance telephone conversation with an energy healer who encouraged me to try quartz crystal bowls.

## QUARTZ POWER:
## THE PROPERTIES OF CRYSTAL BOWLS

Many stories have been told about the mythic lost continent of Atlantis, the ancient, fabled civilization that was supposed to have flourished for some 100,000 years, beginning in 150,000 B.C.E. Atlantis is said to have been an extremely sophisticated culture, its citizens possessed of a highly developed knowledge of science and technology as well as the healing arts. Among the tales I've read about Atlanteans is that they traveled by "flying ships," which were fueled with solar energy that had been transformed into a power source by specially cut quartz crystals.

According to the myth of Atlantis, crystals were an integral part of Atlantis's progressive approach to diagnosing and treating ill health. Patients were brought to a special room in the temple that was built of crystal, where diffused solar energy was used to heal, not the physical body, but the "etheric" or energetic body that surrounds the physical body and holds the disease.

The temple priests also used bowl-shaped vessels made of quartz crystal to treat the sick. According to one legend of Atlantis, a High Priest discovered that that the sound vibrations emitted by his bowls could cure various conditions, ranging from emotional distress and imbalance to headaches and sore throats.

"As the bowl was sounded, the pure note rang clearly, and was felt in waves in the body.... It was very peacemaking. He [the High Priest] experimented and found three gongs were right for some, while others, not being quite as sick, needed only one or two."

Although the people of Atlantis were highly evolved, both spiritually and intellectually, there were many who ultimately debased their knowledge to further their own selfish goals. A select group of righteous citizens foresaw the inevitable and left Atlantis, taking with them the secrets of the crystals. The rest of the civilization was destroyed through a series of calamitous earthquakes and floods, visited upon them by the Creator as punishment for their corruption of power.

We don't have to believe in the lore of Atlantis to grasp the significance of its mythology. For many hundreds of years, people have accepted the complex properties of quartz crystals. Today, scientists and healers alike acknowledge the particular characteristics of quartz. In *Vibrational Medicine,* Richard Gerber, M.D., writes about the scientifically based electronic uses of quartz crystal, which provide a window into its potential healing properties. When electric current is applied to quartz crystal, it will induce mechanical movement, and since each plate of quartz has a unique resonant frequency, says Gerber, "the charges oscillate back and forth at the resonant frequency of the crystal." Gerber says that this phenomenon is the basis for crystal oscillator components used in electronic systems and computer chips to generate and maintain specific energy frequencies.

The same phenomenon appears to be the reason for using quartz crystals to generate and maintain energy frequencies in the human body-mind system. Moreover, proponents of therapeutic touch and energy healing believe that crystals "absorb" human energies and feed back those energies in an altered form. Gerber explains:

"The crystalline structure will respond in unique and precise ways to a wide spectrum of energies including heat, light, pressure, sound, electricity, gamma rays, microwaves, bioelectricity, and even the energies of consciousness (i.e., thought waves or thoughtforms.). In response to these varying energetic inputs, the molecular structure of the crystal will undergo particular modes of oscillation, thereby creating specific vibratory frequencies of energy emission."

These vibratory frequencies of energy emission may explain the healing properties of quartz crystals as used by psychic and medicinal healers, whether they are Native American shamans or New Age practitioners. As Michael Harner explains, "The tribal shamans of cultures throughout the world have quartz crystals among their collections of power objects. In such widely separated peoples as the Jivaro in South America and the tribes of Australia, the quartz crystal is considered the strongest power object of all."

While I can't comment on the healing properties of quartz crystals in this context, Marcel Vogel, who worked as a senior scientist at IBM for nearly three decades and has spent many years researching quartz crystals, has concluded that "the crystal emits a vibration which extends and amplifies the powers of the user's mind. Like a laser, it radiates energy in a coherent, highly concentrated form, and this energy may be transmitted into objects or people at will."

If we accept Vogel's premise, it seems that quartz crystals can be used in a variety of ways to absorb and transmit varying patterns of energy with equally varying effects on mind and body. As Gerber points out, the crystalline structure will respond in unique and precise ways to a spectrum of energies, including sound. Quartz crystal bowls vibrate at frequencies that produce powerful sound waves, and these sounds are the energetic manifestation of the crystalline structure of the bowls themselves.

Thus, the bowl sound may resonate in a uniquely harmonious fashion with the human body, since, as Marcel Vogel says, our healthy human tissues are more crystalline than fluid in nature. Moreover, the framework of bone and collagen is partly comprised of calcium phosphate crystal. All these crystals must have a "resonation potential," and no doubt the sounds produced by quartz crystal are more harmoniously in tune with our own crystalline structures than sounds emitted by other bowls or instruments. Given the other properties of crystal, namely its apparent absorption and emission of energies that both reflect and influence human consciousness, the special properties of quartz crystal bowls should come as no surprise.

While aspects of this theory are speculative, my patients' as well as my own experiences with quartz crystal bowls strongly support the hypothesis that the overtones they produce have resonant and healing properties unlike anything we have encountered. The bowls emit tones that resonate with the human voice. The sounds permeate our systems, resonating with our essence, so that inner chaos, conflict, and dissonance seem almost immediately to be transformed into harmony.

## CRYSTAL BOWLS AND BODY-MIND HEALING

My meeting with Ödsal was a life-changing encounter. As I discovered the power of sound, my own spiritual and emotional growth accelerated rapidly, which served to confirm my belief that I had more to offer my patients than routine medical diagnosis and treatment. I had already started to introduce various breathing and guided imagery techniques as a way to reduce stress, but the bowls represented a whole new dimension in healing that was simply too exciting not to share with anyone who was willing to listen.

Given the choice between a doctor who is a superb technician and a doctor who is also a healer, most people who are ill or in pain will gravitate toward the latter. I also suspect that most doctors are searching for satisfaction and fulfillment—and the only way they can achieve those goals is to become healers themselves, because each time we bring healing energy to someone, a part of us is also healed. Of course, it doesn't require a medical degree to be a healer, in its broadest definition. We simply need to become attuned to the very delicate vibrations of the universe, because once we resonate with our true essence, we cannot help but become more loving, more intuitive, more capable of reacting from our most open and compassionate self.

I cannot, however, draw you a diagram or offer you an easy-to-follow, step-by-step technique that will help you find your true essence. What I can do is provide a kind of spiritual road map. Think of the bowls, not as an end in themselves, but rather as a vehicle, with you as the driver. You want to follow this map, knowing that you're headed in the right direction, moving toward the infinite, toward absolute creativity, toward absolute love. There is no final destination. There is only the continuous becoming, the constantly evolving into your truest self.

The bowls demonstrate the truly manifold possibilities for healing through vibratory sound. The principle of entrainment explains these possibilities; our body-mind systems are "retuned" by the bowl sounds, and the effects can be physical, psychological, spiritual, or all three at once.

I speak from personal experience. I am not the same person I was before I started using the bowls during my meditation practice. Like most people, I was accustomed to seeing the world purely from the limited perspective of my personal awareness. I had to deal with the same stress that all doctors confront. Through my practice with the bowls, I became more in touch with my essence. If I was holding on to a stressful feeling or thought, all I had to do was play one of my bowls, and that feeling or thought would be transformed. I grew more compassionate, more creative in terms of being able to heal, in being able to build my life as I want to live it.

I also speak from my experiences with my patients. I experimented with playing the bowls while they were undergoing chemotherapy and saw their anxiety dissipate as they submerged themselves in the sounds. I played the bowls for people in my office and during my support groups and watched them take extraordinary emotional, physical, and spiritual leaps forward.

Rachel became my patient when she came to see me for a second opinion after she was diagnosed at age forty-eight with metastatic breast cancer. Her oncologist had informed her she needed chemotherapy, but Rachel was insistent that I come up with an alternative. "No chemo," she declared. "I'm not doing it, no matter what."

I agreed with her doctor, and I said so, but her tone was so resolute that I didn't become argumentative. Instead, hoping to discover what lay behind her opposition to the appropriate treatment, I asked her about her family background. She told me that her parents had fled Europe for the United States just before World War II; they alone of their families had survived the Holocaust. Their marriage was an unhappy one: Her father was a cold, distant man who used any excuse to stay away from home. Her mother, who had severe emotional problems, used Rachel as a go-between to communicate with her father. "Go ask him why he didn't get back until two in the morning," she would typically instruct Rachel. "Find out when he plans to come back tonight."

Rachel's words came haltingly, as if she hardly knew how to speak about the long-ago circumstances that still ruled her life. It became clear to me that from a very early age, Rachel had sympathized with her father's need to avoid her mother. At the same time, however, she had identified with her mother's anguish and confusion. The conflicting feelings were too much for the young girl to carry. Growing up with a remote, withdrawn father and an utterly self-absorbed mother, neither of whom could give her any love, Rachel came to the conclusion that she was unlovable. Her solution was to shut down, to close off her heart rather than consciously feel the pain her parents unwittingly inflicted upon her.

"I've never discussed this before, not even with my husband," she said, suddenly interrupting herself. "I didn't think anyone would care enough to listen." She thanked me for giving her this opportunity, then smiled grimly. "But I still won't do chemotherapy."

I said I understood and recommended that she attend the upcoming meeting of my bimonthly support group, if only to get a taste of the stress reduction techniques I practice there with my patients. I didn't have much hope that she would actually show up, so I was surprised when I walked into the conference room two nights later and saw her seated at the table with the other participants.

As I normally do, I began by inviting people to talk about any feelings or thoughts that had come up for them since our last meeting. Rachel was silent throughout the discussion, and when I asked for volunteers to lie down on the floor one at a time so that I could place around them Tibetan and crystal bowls and "bathe" them in sound (as I did with my brother-in-law, Keith), she almost squirmed with discomfort. But after watching—and listening to—a demonstration, Rachel put up her hand. She was ready to try this out for herself.

In the course of using the bowls to work with hundreds of patients, I've witnessed many reactions, many transformations. But few have been quite so dramatic as what I saw happen that evening for Rachel. She seemed nervous at first, although less than I might have expected her to be. But the change that took place as the sound waves moved through and around her was as profound as it was immediately apparent. The smile on her face was so sweet and innocent that I felt as if she had traveled back to a moment in her childhood before she had unconsciously adopted the belief that she didn't deserve to be loved.

Immersed in the vibrations of the bowls, she was hearing for

## Meditating with a Mantra

Find a comfortable place to sit, either in a straight-backed chair or cross-legged on a mat or pillow. Make sure that you won't be disturbed for the next fifteen minutes: Close your door and, if necessary, hang a Do Not Disturb sign on the knob. Turn off the telephone and answering machine. Before you begin, choose as your mantra a simple word or meaningful phrase that can help you maintain your focus. You might try using the Sanskrit mantra *Ham Sah,* which means "I am that," breathing in on *"Ham,"* and out on *"Sah."* Once you've decided on a mantra, close your eyes and practice either of the two breathing exercises I described in Chapter Two. When you feel that your breathing has slowed and deepened, start to concentrate on thinking *"Ham"* (or whatever word or phrase you've chosen) as you inhale, and *"Sah"* when you exhale. Inhale and exhale through your nose, in a silent, threadlike breath.

Don't get discouraged if your attention begins to wander—and it will. If you notice a pain in your neck or back, or your nose itches, or your foot feels as if it's falling asleep, try to stay still and maintain your posture. But don't feel as if you're failing some sort of test if you have to adjust your position or scratch your nose. This is all part of learning how to meditate.

Each time you realize that you've stopped concentrating on your mantra, and your mind has turned instead to your grocery list, the work you left unfinished on your desk, an unresolved argument with your husband or wife, or any other emotionally engaging thought, bring your attention back to your breath and your mantra. Are you inhaling fully and exhaling slowly? Pause after every inhalation and exhalation, slowing the rhythm of your breath so that your lungs and abdomen fully expand and contract.

Be compassionate with yourself. The practice of meditation requires patience and commitment. When distractions appear on the screen that is your mind, notice them, then let them go. Refocus your awareness on your mantra and breathing.

Start the meditation practice by setting aside ten to twenty minutes for each session. (You may want to keep a watch or clock nearby.) As the end of your meditation draws near, gradually begin to become aware of your surroundings and how you are feeling. Open your eyes slowly and allow yourself as much time as you need before you open the door and reimmerse yourself in your daily schedule.

the first time in her life the absolute beauty and harmony of the universe—the subtle sounds of her own essence. This unconditional harmony, which can only come from within, empowered Rachel to see herself as someone who deserved to get better, someone who could be vulnerable and accept help.

I don't mean to imply that all of her issues were resolved after a single exposure to the sounds of the bowls. But every one of us in that room was aware that an important shift in her energy had taken place. Rachel's healing—spiritual, emotional, and physical—started that evening. Shortly thereafter, she purchased her own crystal bowl and used it in conjunction with her newly established meditation practice. As she grew more in touch with her essence, she stopped looking at herself as a limited, ego-based, body-centered organism and found instead her connection with the divine infinite. She also continued exploring the childhood issues that were still having such a strong impact on her life. She overcame her fears about chemotherapy and agreed to undergo a course of treatment, the side effects of which turned out to be far less difficult than she'd imagined them to be. And when the chemotherapy regimen failed to produce the hoped-for results, Rachel unhesitatingly agreed to undergo a bone marrow transplant, a physically and emotionally demanding procedure that she previously would never have considered. Two years later, Rachel is in remission from her cancer. She attends my support group as often as she can and maintains her spiritual practice that, she tells me, strengthens her resolve to survive and enriches every aspect of her life.

The sound of the bowls, and the way in which those sounds resonated within her, served as a reminder to Rachel that she was much more than her illness, or her negative childhood history, or the distorted self-image she'd carried with her into adulthood. Her work with the bowls helped her rediscover her essence, her connection to the infinite. This reawakened awareness enabled her to abandon the harsh, critical lens through which she viewed herself and the world, to find self-esteem in a far broader "Self" than the wounded, ego-based one she'd always identified with. How important was this metamorphosis? Not only did it represent a spiritual awakening for Rachel, it enabled her to choose life-saving medical treatment.

Rachel had no previous experience with meditation, so I taught her the fundamental technique, Meditating with a Mantra, which is the starting point for many mind-body practices, including those that involve sound.

## WRITING YOUR OWN LIFE SONG

Legend has it that when Buddha was asked, "What did you do before you achieved enlightenment?" he answered, "I chopped wood and carried water." The next question posed was: "And now that you have achieved enlightenment?" Buddha replied, "I chop wood and carry water."

On the most mundane, day-to-day level, nothing had changed. Yet everything was different, because his point of view had radically altered. It is precisely this shift in perspective that I encourage my patients to explore through sound-centered meditation.

The shift occurs far more rapidly and powerfully when the bowl sounds are combined with unique forms of vocal expression. In my work on myself and my patients, I've developed a method, based in part on Native American, Tibetan, Hindu, and other vocal practices of the great wisdom traditions, in which we create and sing what I prefer to call our "life song."

These songs are mantralike sounds, comprised of groups of syllables strung together in a pattern that is as unique to you as your social security number. Life songs transform our jumbled thoughts, judgments, and feelings into a harmonious pattern. Chanting our life song while we play the bowls allows the clatter of what Zen Buddhists call "monkey mind" to recede into the background, thus making room for an expansive consciousness through which we can find our essence.

Consider the case of Gordon, a high-powered television network executive whose mind never stopped its feverish activity. Gordon's already skyrocketing stress levels went through the roof when I told him that he'd relapsed for the fourth time with non-Hodgkin's lymphoma. "My father died recently," he told me. "But I just turned forty-four. I'm not ready to go yet."

My intuition told me that Gordon was repressing some very strong, painful emotions that could interfere with his recovery. He'd never spoken of his father before, and when I asked him to talk about his death, Gordon surprised himself—and me—by bursting into tears. Normally composed and reticent, Gordon suddenly let the words tumble out of him like a torrent of water rushing downstream.

He was more relieved than grief-stricken that his father had passed away, he told me. His father had been a driven, competitive man whose wife had had to be institutionalized with severe postpartum depression immediately after the birth of their only child. The father had blamed the boy for his mother's breakdown, and he'd punished him by insisting that Gordon participate in and excel at team sports, whether or not he was interested in playing any of them.

By the time he reached adulthood, Gordon's unconscious, unexpressed rage was so all-consuming that it was literally killing him. Like his father, he saw life as a competitive game, and not one that yielded much pleasure. Though he had a loving family, his relationships were not a source of much emotional gratification. I saw my task as twofold: to prescribe the correct course of therapy that would treat Gordon's lymphoma, and to help him reconnect with his essence so that he could heal the wounds inflicted by his father, transcend his rage, and reestablish loving ties with family and friends.

I invited Gordon to attend my support group, and I also suggested that he immediately begin the healing process by "writing" his life song. (Instructions on how to write your life song appear on the following pages.)

Under other circumstances, Gordon probably would have dismissed my request as "new age nonsense." But knowing that he faced a life-and-death situation, he was willing to try just about anything. I won't reveal the particular grouping of syllables he chose, since like mantras, they should remain private and personal. Suffice it to say that Gordon found a life song he could vocalize with the bowls, one that brought joy into his heart where before there had been only fury, confusion, and sorrow.

As I write this, Gordon has been in remission from his recurrent lymphoma for eleven months after an intensive chemotherapy regimen. My fervent hope is that he will continue to be cancer-free. But whatever the ultimate course of his disease, I know that doing the hard work of personal transformation, with the help of sound healing and most especially his life song, has given Gordon a quality of life he had never imagined possible.

I encourage you to create your own life song. Keep in mind, however, that the goal is not to "do it right," but rather to find a string of primal sounds that resonates within you as a profound

## Creating Your Life Song

| RHYMES WITH "HOME" | RHYMES WITH "MOM" |
|---|---|
| HOME | HAM |
| ROME | RAM |
| SOME | SAM |
| LOME | LAM |
| VOME | VAM |
| YOME | YAM |

| RHYMES WITH "KNEE" | RHYMES WITH "HUM" |
|---|---|
| HEE | HUM |
| REE | RUM |
| SEE | SUM |
| LEE | LUM |
| VEE | VUM |
| YEE | YUM |

RHYMES WITH "BLUE"

HOO
ROO
SOO
LOO
NOO

1. Pronounce each of the mantra sounds listed above at the same time that you tap your bowl or listen to a tape of pure sounds. Try them in one order, then another. Keeping your eyes open, say each sound aloud each time you gently strike the bowl.
2. After you complete the entire list, begin to play the bowl by tapping the rim gently three times and applying the mallet clockwise around the rim with firm but gentle pressure. Do not let the bowl begin to vibrate or the sound to become too loud, as the bowl may crack.

(continued on page 126)

(continued from page 125)

3. As you maintain a soft, sustained tone, close your eyes and allow the sounds to come into your mind. Mentally play with the different sounds in various sequences, until you find the combination that most resonates within you. Begin to sing these sounds aloud, using whatever melody comes to you. If no particular melody occurs to you, simply chant the sounds in whichever order feels right. You will most likely find your melody later. Choose three or four sounds that most appeal to you. The sounds that feel the most harmonious to you make up your life song. Examples of a life song might be: SOM MA TUM, LAM MA TOM, TA KEY LA, or TA ME HUM.

The first life song you discover may be the only one you will ever use. On the other hand, you may discover a new song after several weeks, months, or years as you progress along your healing path. There is no "right" or "wrong" life song. Experiment with the sounds as much and as often as you like in all their various combinations. As you chant your life song, you will begin to feel it literally flowing out of you, as if your essence, rather than you yourself, were singing. Allow any subtle changes in the sounds or melody to occur, so that the song remains natural and fluid.

Remember: Your life song is unique and belongs only to you. It can connect you with your essence whenever you chant it, either aloud or silently. I therefore recommend that you respect your song by keeping it private. Many people, myself included, find that chanting our life song silently when we are in stressful situations gives us great inner peace and strength.

expression of who you are. If you own or have access to a bowl, use the sounds of the bowl to guide you in composing your life song. Otherwise, ignore the instructions in steps 1 and 2 about how to incorporate the bowls, and simply chant the sounds aloud as you experiment with them. The sounds listed are offered as suggestions to get you started, but feel free to invent your own sounds made up of any combination of vowels and consonants. Permit yourself to be as a creative, uninhibited, and playful as a young child throughout this process.

# PART II

# TUNING MIND, BODY, AND SOUL

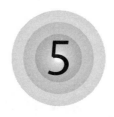

## 5

SOUND BODY:

# Recovery and Total Wellness

Sandy, a tenacious young woman who was diagnosed last year with breast cancer, recently recalled for me how discouraged she felt when she met with her oncologist after she'd had a mastectomy. "I always knew I was a pretty resilient person, and I have very strong willpower," she said. "Even when I heard that the cancer was stage III, which wasn't a great situation, I figured I could do things that other people couldn't."

The stage III classification refers to a large breast tumor that has spread to nearby lymph nodes in the armpit but is not detectable elsewhere in the body. Lymph node involvement means that microscopic cancer has likely escaped into the body and will eventually appear as a potentially lethal metastatic tumor, unless chemotherapy and/or the patient's immune system can effectively eliminate the wayward cells.

In my experience, state-of-the-art chemotherapy in conjunction with nutritional and mind-body medicine can be used to vastly improve survival rates for women in Sandy's predicament. Moreover, Sandy, a veteran marathoner, had completed a five-mile run just four days after surgery. "I thought, wow! I feel pretty good," she said. But her upbeat attitude quickly dissipated in the face of her doctor's pronouncement that the follow-up chemotherapy, for which she was already scheduled, would reduce her chance of a recurrence by only a few percentage points.

Sandy was referred to me by a friend because she wanted a second opinion from a doctor who practiced a holistic approach to cancer prevention and treatment. She was visibly relieved when I told her that I recommended chemotherapy in combination with a low-fat, high-fiber diet, nutritional supplements, sound-based meditation, and visualization as her many weapons to prevent the cancer from returning. Initially dubious about the role that emotional factors played in affecting her health, Sandy nevertheless joined my support group.

"I knew I had to stop ignoring my emotional issues, because I was feeling depressed and really scared," she said. "I thought that meeting other people might be a good thing, and I'd read that women with breast cancer who joined support groups lived a lot longer."

Sandy had never meditated before, and she describes her first experience as "a bit unnerving. It took me a while to feel comfortable about closing my eyes in a room full of strangers, trying to block everything out so I could focus on my breath and the sound of the bowl. Afterward, I liked how I felt, so I kept coming to the meetings, even on days when I had my chemo treatment."

Sandy calls me her cheerleader, because I informed her at our first appointment that I'd treated hundreds of women who hadn't had recurrences. "You told me then, 'I know you can get through it!' And that's what I wanted to hear," she reminded me the last time we spoke. "Because if your doctor doesn't believe that you can overcome it, how can you?"

I, too, believe that creating a "healing partnership" between doctor and patient has vital therapeutic value. But Sandy deserves the credit for taking charge of her future by deciding to beat her disease with all the resources at her command. Her resiliency is an excellent example of what Steven Greer, M.D., defined as "fighting spirit." In his research at the Royal Marsden Hospital near London, Dr. Greer and his colleagues showed that breast cancer patients with fighting spirit—those who believed that their proactive attitude and actions would vastly improve their chances for recovery—were twice as likely to have survived over fifteen years than patients who felt helpless and hopeless.

Despite her initial reservations, Sandy discovered that sound meditation and guided imagery were extremely useful techniques to help her deal with the rigors of chemotherapy as well as a demanding job as a commercial real estate agent. "I'm never going to get to the point where I don't have stress," she says. "But it bothers me less, and I'm able to reduce the level much more quickly and effectively because of these tools." She describes the sounds of the bowls as "very powerful. The vibrations bring me into a calm state more easily than when I meditate on my own. All the stress and distractions just fade away."

This past summer, Sandy realized a longtime fantasy when she spent a week hiking in the French Alps, a strenuous vacation by anyone's standards. She is currently undergoing her final round of chemotherapy, and her current health and future prognosis are excellent. Sandy maintains a four-mile-a-day running routine, and she and I remain convinced that her energy and optimism will help fend off any recurrences.

Sandy's experience exemplifies how sound and meditation may influence health and healing, in part through the mechanism of the mind-body connection. I believe that all physical illness is a manifestation of a mind-body imbalance that extends even to the cellular level. In Chapter Two, I discussed mind-body research that confirms the havoc that chronic negative emotions can wreak on our various physiologic systems, leading to serious health problems—unless we take steps to release the emotions and change the patterns.

For instance, you may fail to notice that you carry stress in your neck until you develop a stiff neck. A heating pad and aspirins temporarily cure the condition, but the symptoms inevitably return. Soon you begin to suffer from serious pain in your back, and when you consult your doctor, you're told that you've developed a herniated disk. Untreated, the disk could cause you to lose the use of an arm; surgery is recommended.

But what if we looked beyond the symptoms and the ailment—whether it's a stiff neck or an ulcer, cancer or heart disease—to determine the emotional source of the physiologic disharmony? What if we finally tapped the extraordinary ability of the mind to heal our gravest pains?

Years before scientists had ever thought to research the relationship between mind and body, let alone the influence of sound on either, Sufi master Hazrat Inayat Khan wrote, "The physical effect of sound has also a great influence upon the human body. The whole mechanism, the muscles, the blood circulation, the nerves are all moved by the power of vibration. As there is resonance for every sound, so the human body is a living resonator for sound. . . . Every pitch that is a natural pitch of the voice will be a source of a person's own healing as well as of that of others when he sings a note of that pitch." The power of the mind to correct physiologic imbalances is no longer the revolutionary idea it was once considered to be, but the use of sound and music to harness that power is only now being explored.

## SOUND HEALING: THE CELLULAR BRIDGE

Sound enters the healing equation from several directions: It may alter cellular functions through energetic effects; it may entrain biological systems to function more homeostatically; it may becalm the mind and therefore the body; or it may have emotional effects, which influence neurotransmitters and neuropeptides, which in turn help to regulate the immune system—the healer within. Music, of course, is organized sound that has potent emotional effects and stimulates memories, associations, and highly developed psychological states with clear impact on our healing systems.

As I mentioned earlier, Beverly Rubik, a leading synthesizer of research on energy medicine, suggests that electromagnetic energy, and perhaps other forms of energy, influence cellular function at the level of the cell receptor. Candace Pert has pointed out that cell receptors, which receive biological "information" from neuropeptides, neurotransmitters, and other molecular messengers, "change shape, shimmy, and even hum." Remember, how receptors react to molecular messengers (whether and how they change shape) can help determine the actions of our immune defender cells and virtually every other cell in the body.

Perhaps the most scientifically sophisticated work on the effects of various types of energy on cellular function comes from the laboratory of biophysicist Jan Walleczek at the Loma Linda Veterans Administration Medical Center in California. Walleczek has proven that Extremely Low Frequency (ELF) electromagnetic fields trigger cellular changes, particularly on T-lymphocytes, the soldier cells of the immune system. Walleczek has published many studies in peer-reviewed journals showing that ELF fields can either stimulate or inhibit the action of immune cells, depending in part on the level of exposure.

Walleczek is looking at how ELF energy fields influence cellular actions, and his experiments suggest that they do so by regulating the uptake of calcium. Specifically, these fields influence the release of intracellular stores of calcium, the entry of calcium into cells, and the enzyme systems that also control the cellular dynamics of calcium uptake. In one of his provocative papers, Walleczek also points out that DNA synthesis may be calcium dependent, and may therefore be influenced by energy fields.

What does this suggest about the effect of sound on cell

function? Sound is certainly a form of energy, although not identical with the ELF energy fields studied by Walleczek. Other researchers, including Fabien Maman, a French composer and bio-energeticist, have begun to explore and document the specific influence on cells of sound wave energies. Maman's dual interest in music and such energy-based healing techniques as acupuncture led him to wonder: "Are we really touched and even changed by music? If so, how deeply does sound travel in the body?" In 1981 he teamed up with Helene Grimal, a biologist at the French National Center for Scientific Research in Paris; for a year and a half, he and Grimal examined through microscopic photography the effect of low frequency (30–40 decibels) sound on human cells. In Maman's words, "The goal of these experiments was to observe the effect of sound in the nucleus and the electromagnetic fields of human cells."

Using a camera mounted on a microscope, Maman and Grimal studied the inner structure of both healthy human cells and uterine cancer cells as they reacted to various acoustical instruments, e.g., gong, xylophone, acoustic guitar, and the unaccompanied human voice, for a duration of twenty-one minutes.

Maman found that the most visibly dramatic results occurred when he sang musical scales into the cells: "The structure disorganized extremely quickly. The human voice carries something in its vibration that makes it more powerful than any musical instrument: consciousness. . . . It appeared that the cancer cells were not able to support a progressive accumulation of vibratory frequencies. As soon as I introduced the third frequency in the sequence, the cells began to destabilize." But the other instruments, particularly the gong with its rich complement of overtones, also caused the cells to disintegrate and ultimately explode.

Based upon his findings within the laboratory, Maman then conducted experiments with two breast cancer patients, each of whom toned for three and a half hours a day over the course of a month. In one case, the tumor vanished. The second woman had surgery to remove the tumor, whereupon it was discovered that the tumor was "reduced and completely dry." In the absence of metastases, the malignancy was excised and the patient made a full recovery.

In his book *The Role of Music in the Twenty-first Century,* Maman includes fascinating photographs—some taken with an ordinary camera and some with a Kirlian photographic machine that records electromagnetic fields—that graphically illustrate the reactions of the cells. He writes:

> This finding indicates that the vibration of sound plays a determinant role in the transformation of cellular structure, acting directly at the most subtle level of the human organism. . . . As long as we played the whole chromatic musical scale for the same length of time, different levels of energy were stimulated at the same time and the diseased cell was too disrupted to stabilize. The addition of the vibratory rate became too powerful and the cell could not adapt to it. The cell died because it was not able to accommodate its structure and synchronize with the accumulation of sound.

Maman also collaborated with French physicist Joel Sternheimer, who reported in his article "The Music of the Elementary Particles" his discovery that every human molecule has a particular corresponding musical frequency. "The masses of particles behave and maneuver among themselves as if they were musical notes on the chromatic tempered scale," Sternheimer noted. Thus, concludes Maman, the explosions within the cells may be caused by the dissonance between the frequencies of the particles within the cell structure and the sound vibrations.

Maman's provocative photographs of cancer cells show evidence of cell nuclei incapable of maintaining their structure as the sound wave frequencies "attack" the cytoplasmic and nuclear membranes. His experiments echo the much earlier investigations of Ernst Chladni, a seventeenth-century German scientist and amateur musician, who has been called the "father of acoustics." Chladni thrilled French scientists and Napoleon himself in 1809 when he proved his thesis that sound vibrations could move matter, by sprinkling sand atop a plate affixed to a pedestal, then drawing a violin bow around the circumference of the plate, thereby rearranging the sand into intricately patterned geometric designs.

The late Swiss scientist Dr. Hans Jenny used twentieth-century technology to refine and expand upon Chladni's experiments; he named this scientific study of how sound affects matter *cymatics,* after the Greek word for "wave." Jenny used crystal oscillators and the tonoscope, a machine he invented that produced pictures of the human voice, to create stunningly complex forms out of sand and other materials, including iron filings, fine-grained plastic, and mercury. The shape of the designs thus created are infinitely varied, depending on the frequency, amplitude, and type of material, and often resemble exquisite kaleidoscopic configurations with three-dimensional depth and texture, some of which mimic naturally occurring universal forms, such as snowflakes, flowers, and spirals.

I was especially fascinated to learn that chanting the mantra *OM* produces a series of interlayered concentric diamonds and triangles set within a perfect circle, an image strikingly similar to the Tantric Buddhist mandala that represents the sacred pulsations of creation.

But my interest was truly piqued when I read that Jenny, who chronicled his life work in *Cymatics,* and in a movie of the same name, theorized that each human cell has its own frequency, and that the frequency of every human organ may be a harmonic of its component cells. Thus, we are offered the intriguing hypothesis that these signature frequencies hold the key to unlocking the mystery of how sound can be used to heal on the cellular and genetic levels. Sir Peter Guy Manners, M.D., an English osteopath, has researched and developed a clinical application of Jenny's theories, known as "cymatic therapy," which involves using audible sound waves to stimulate overlapping biological systems, including the immune system, in order to achieve a near-ideal metabolic state in a cell or organ.

Manners views disease as "an interruption of an organ's harmonious molecular relationship." He uses cymatic therapy not to cure a particular condition, but rather to help the body heal itself by promoting a state of chemical and homeostatic balance.

> By intercepting the electrical messages transmitted via the central nervous system to individual cells, this research has allowed the coding of cymatic signals that cells understand. Each tissue has been given an H-factor (harmonic factor) according to the signal emitted. The cymatic instrument adjusts acoustic audible sound frequencies in order to induce beneficial stimulation, activation, and circulation when applied to the body via direct contact with affected areas or by way of acupuncture meridians.

Cymatic therapy, which was introduced into the United States some thirty years ago, has been used to treat rheumatism, paralysis, muscle strain, arthritis, bone fracture, and various other conditions. Manners hopes that it also may be used in the future for organ transplantation, to help create resonance between the transplanted organ and the recipient, and to encourage regeneration in the peripheral nerves, bones, and skin.

## Bowls, Brain Waves, and the Rings of Uranus

The findings of Fabien Maman and cymatic therapy someday could have direct repercussions for people with cancer and other diseases of cellular degeneration or dysfunction. A related but even more sophisticated approach is now being investigated by Jeffrey Thompson, D.C., who directs the Center for Neuroacoustic Research at the California Institute for Human Science. Thompson practices a technique he calls "Sonic Induction Therapy," which involves the use of sound frequency vibrations to promote balance in various biological systems and even to stimulate cellular healing.

Thompson creates an acoustical mix of electronically disguised sounds from nature—birds, dolphins, human voices, waves, wind, and other "organic" tones—that he calls a "primordial sound"; this sound, he says, resonates and entrains patients' brain waves and other physiologic functions, prompting profound relaxation and a "state of subconscious openness." He also uses ingenious sonic technologies to uncover and reproduce his patients' fundamental sound frequency—their vocal fingerprints, so to speak. Thompson believes he can tap into the unique harmonics and overtones of an individual's voiceprint in order to rectify imbalances at both subconscious and cellular levels.

The voiceprint is created from modified 3–D recordings of the patient's own voice, delivered through a custom-designed sound therapy table with "tuning fork" transducers that turn the entire table into a giant vibrational sounding board. According to Thompson, "Part of the reason for the profound responses experienced by some people . . . is a result of direct cellular vibration with this sound table."

Thompson is convinced that sound delivered at the proper frequency range and vibrational intensity can, at least theoretically, heal at the cellular level:

"Since the human body is over seventy percent water and since sound travels five times more efficiently through water than through air, sound frequency stimulation directly into the body is a highly efficient means for total body stimulation, especially at the cellular level. Direct stimulation of living cellular tissue using sound frequency vibration has shown marked cellular metabolism and therefore a possible mobilization of a cellular healing response."

Thompson's "bio-tuning" and sound induction techniques—which draw upon every variety of sound found in nature for his psychoacoustic interventions—are certainly among the most sophisticated new approaches to sound healing. His recordings of disguised primordial sounds prompted a phone call from a NASA official who had heard Thompson's audiotapes. The official asked whether Thompson had listened to any of the *Voyager I* or *II* spacecraft recordings from deep space, because some of them sounded precisely like Thompson's own nature recordings.

Thompson was not surprised to discover that the sounds recorded in outer space were, indeed, strikingly similar to natural sonic emissions reproduced in his own recordings. For instance, sounds emitted by the planet Jupiter markedly resemble the high-pitched cries of dolphins, and sounds from the smallest moon of Uranus (Miranda) resemble vocal choirs. But Thompson was most intrigued by the sounds produced by the rings of Uranus, which are virtually identical to those produced by Tibetan bowls.

Thompson believes that this similarity is no coincidence; he sees both as sonic reverberations of what Carl Jung described as the collective unconscious, reminding us on cellular and spiritual levels of our primordial roots. "If one travels deep enough into the subconscious, one eventually reaches a level . . . common to all people," says Thompson. Perhaps the reverberations of Tibetan and crystal bowls are powerfully healing precisely because they are so similar to primordial space sounds, the sound of our cosmic essence.

Early in his career as a chiropractor seeking more effective treatments for chronic back pain and other musculoskeletal disorders, Thompson wondered whether sound vibrations could promote alignment and healing. He reports that he's achieved excellent results in the treatment of dyslexia, attention deficit disorders, and certain learning disabilities.

One clinically measured physiologic effect of his sound interventions is the altering of brain waves into alpha and theta frequency ranges, which according to many EEG biofeedback experts represent mind/brain states of relaxation and heightened receptivity to healing. But is there evidence that changing brain waves via sound therapy can have clinically meaningful effects on health?

Specialists in EEG biofeedback (also known as neurofeedback) help people modify their own brain wave patterns and have documented improvements in a laundry list of conditions, from attention deficit disorder to stroke to hypertension. But perhaps the most compelling recent work illuminates a link between brain wave adjustments and a stronger immune system. Gary Schummer, Ph.D., of the Pacific Institute for Behavioral Medicine, has conducted studies showing that HIV patients who regularly use EEG biofeedback to achieve alpha and theta brain wave states experience statistically significant increases in their T-helper cells—a crucial indicator of the ability to stave off full-blown AIDS. When this work is considered in the context of Dr. Thompson's research on sound and brain wave entrainment, we begin to see how sound may influence the brain-body nexus, which even encompasses our immune defense network.

Thompson's work also sheds light on the healing properties of Tibetan and crystal bowl sounds. An increasing number of mind-body practitioners appear to be using the bowls to bolster the recovery process for a wide range of physical conditions and diseases. Con Potanin, M.D., the medical director of the Mind-Body Institute at Baptist Hospital in Nashville, Tennessee, combines chanting and music with Tibetan and crystal bowls for patients who suffer from chronic pain problems that include migraine headaches; neck, shoulder, and back pain; hypertension; and irritable bowel syndrome.

Potanin finds the blending of Tibetan bowls and music works most effectively when used within the context of a group. "This helps to de-stress them so that they're capable of doing meditation and relaxation exercises that sometimes include stretching and yoga," he says. He is quick to add, however, that the meditation is not an end in itself, but rather a means by which to arrive at "spiritual aspects like forgiveness. The meditation opens up the mind and enables patients to address the part that fear and anger have played in their problems."

Potanin's experience using crystal and Tibetan bowls for pain management and stress-related disorders, and my own experience with cancer and other serious diseases, constitute ample anecdotal evidence that these sounds, so rich in harmonic overtones, gently guide the body-mind toward homeostasis and healing.

## SOUND, MUSIC, IMAGERY, AND THE IMMUNE SYSTEM

Clinical psychologist and music therapist Mark Rider, Ph.D., and his colleagues have produced compelling hard data demonstrating that music, when combined with guided imagery, can reduce stress hormones *and* raise levels of disease-fighting immune cells. For example, in one study conducted by Rider, a group of university students was lectured on the secretion of antibodies. They were then instructed to imagine antibody production while listening to live improvised music, which, they were told, would facilitate their imagery. A second group listened to the same music without any other instructions, while a third group sat in silence. At the end of the session, the production of sIgA (secretory immunoglobulin A) antibodies was tested through collection of saliva and measurement of skin temperature. Rider found that sIgA production was significantly higher in the imagery/music group than in either of the other groups.

In another experiment conducted by Rider and Jeanne Achterberg, a leader in the field of psychoneuroimmunology (PNI) and a recognized expert in the uses of imagery for healing, a group of college students listened to a seventeen-minute-long tape with specially composed background music and instructions on how to visualize their B-cells making copious antibodies that fight disease agents. Another group listened to a tape that played only the music, while a control group simply sat in silence for a seventeen-minute period. All three groups were tested for production of sIgA before and after they listened to the tape or (in the case of the control group) sat silently. Rider found that the production of antibodies in Groups 1 and 2 were significantly greater than in the control group, and that after three weeks of training, Group 1 surpassed Group 2, suggesting, says Rider, "that imagery allows for a more advanced type of conditioning of the immune system than is available by relaxation alone."

Remarkably, we seem to be able to directly influence the behavior of specific classes of cells with equally specific mind-pictures. Rider and Achterberg carried out a study in which they divided subjects into two groups, both of which were given six weeks of music-enhanced instruction in how to visualize the activity of two key classes of disease-fighting white blood cells, neutrophils and lymphocytes. "Amazingly, only the blood cell [type] which was focused on changed significantly for both groups, indicating again that an immediate biological effect was able to be communicated to the immune system," Rider comments.

The use of imagery clearly adds a dimension to the healing effects of sound and music, which makes sense, given that imagery has its own independent, positive effect on the immune system. Pioneering work conducted in the mid-'70s by Achterberg, Frank Lawlis, Ph.D., Carl Simonton, Ph.D., and Stephanie Simonton, Ph.D., demonstrated that "imagery of a positive outcome" correlated most highly among psychological and blood chemistry factors with surviving terminal cancer.

What, exactly, is guided imagery? When we visualize images that arouse an emotion, a sense of serenity, or physical sensations, an entire cascade of physiologic changes occur, including modulation of neurotransmitters, neuropeptides, and messenger molecules that may influence the immune system. The process itself is simple: We sit quietly in a meditative state, allowing ourselves to conjure mind-pictures, either from our own imaginations, or from a script or tape or the promptings of a clinician (hence, guided imagery). The psychological and physiological effects of imagery will differ depending on the infinite varieties of visual images we can use, but the power of imagery to change our mind-body state is certain. Consider the simplest example: Close your eyes and imagine yourself sucking on a wedge of lemon. Take your time and really picture the lemon, imagine its texture and taste. Do you notice small jets of saliva under your tongue? You don't need an actual lemon to change your body chemistry, only an imagined one.

The same principle holds when we use imagery to boost the immune system, either directly, by visualizing white blood cells mobilizing for action, killing pathogens and cancer cells; or indirectly, by imagining scenes that produce serenity, which, in turn, reduces stress hormones and bolsters immunity. A world of research in psychoneuroimmunology offers a biological basis for this effect: Brain signals and brain messengers can influence the activity of most subclasses of immune cells. The work of Mark Rider, Jeanne Achterberg, and others suggests that combining music with imagery enhances these effects.

Recently, research has been conducted on the effects of imagery on the immune system that showed the following:

- an increase in natural killer cell activity among healthy subjects using imagery

- increased production of immunoglobulin A (a class of antibodies) among subjects who practiced imagery after *only one training session* that equaled the production by those who practiced relaxation techniques.

- significantly greater activity and numbers of disease-fighting lymphocytes in a subset of healthy volunteers—namely, those younger than fifty—who were given cell-specific imagery instructions. The subjects had been taught self-hypnosis and how to visualize their lymphocytes as powerful sharks swimming through the bloodstream. The improved immune responses were noted after one session, and again after a week of self-hypnosis and imagery practice.

- selective boosting or dampening of the local lymphocyte response to a skin test for varicella zoster. Subjects were able to use imagery to "send a message" to the immune system to either rush to the site of the test, causing a stronger inflammatory response, or to lie back, resulting in far less inflammation.

These experiments with imagery and music represent strong, methodologically tight evidence that we can, to some extent, regulate our immune responses. But the question often arises, rightly, as to whether these immune changes are clinically relevant. Put simply: Do they translate biologically as a meaningful improvement in our ability to fight off disease?

My own clinical experience with countless patients tells me that these biologic changes are indeed meaningful. These patients routinely do better than statistical expectations would predict; they respond more readily to treatments and tend to live longer. One such patient is George, a forty-four-year-old psychiatric social worker who worked at a woman's shelter in the Bronx. George came to see me when his lymphoma recurred after he'd been in remission for four years. The lymphoma was in a moderately advanced stage that required treatment with an aggressive course of chemotherapy in combination with a stem-cell transplant, a procedure that is difficult, risky, and immensely taxing to the patient. The five-year survival rate for stem-cell transplant is extremely variable; one study suggests it may be as low as 30 percent.

Soft-spoken and courteous almost to a fault, George asked me few questions and nodded his head so frequently during our conversation that the gesture seemed more like a nervous tic than a sign of agreement. As I got to know him, I learned that he had few close relationships, and his early, brief marriage had ended in divorce. George had been in psychotherapy for many years, yet he still carried the scars of his abusive childhood. "I grew up believing that the constant threat of verbal, emotional, and physical abuse was totally normal," he told me. "My father would hit me out of the clear blue for no reason. My mother was almost as bad. She would scream at me and blame me for all her problems, including my father. I felt like I had nowhere to turn."

Through therapy, he'd learned that in order to exist—and survive—in his family structure, he'd had to suppress his inner needs and create a persona separate from his true self. Because he'd felt for so long that he had to wear a mask, he ultimately forgot that the mask was only a prop, albeit an important one, and that he was not the person represented by the mask.

George unconsciously perceived himself as despicable, believing he had to have been a horrible child to have deserved such treatment from his parents. He was frequently plagued by nightmares that evoked his childhood fears of severe mistreatment, punishment, and abandonment. Interestingly, when he'd first been diagnosed with lymphoma, the nightmares had stopped and his chronic depression had lifted, then reappeared while he'd been in remission. Now that the lymphoma had recurred, he told me, the bad dreams and negative feelings about himself had mysteriously disappeared again.

I knew that George could benefit greatly from bowl-centered

healing, so I suggested that he work with me to resolve the fears and judgments he'd experienced as a child. His core issue was his severe lack of self-esteem, and over the course of several months of meditation practice and toning, he gave voice to the anguish born of his self-loathing. This helped George become fully cognizant that his child self was suffused with sadness and hopelessness, and thus prevented him from experiencing joy and a sense of connectedness to the universe. He used the sound of the bowls and his voice to move past this contradiction, accepting the child self but transcending its dictates.

As he expanded his awareness of essence, the protective emotional wall that had prevented his enjoyment of life began to disintegrate. He finally permitted himself truly to experience the rage he'd accumulated over a lifetime because of the violence inflicted upon him by his parents. His healing commenced once he'd moved through the rage and was able to see that his parents' cruelty emanated from their own wounded egos.

Over the course of his treatment, he gradually came to a stunning realization: His deeply damaged child self could only feel alive and excited when he felt himself to be at risk of death. Challenged with a life-threatening illness, he responded the way he had as a child: "Once I moved into survival mode, which was the only excitement ever allowed me, I knew I would be OK."

George understood that his unconscious mind was recreating childhood trauma in the form of illness. That is not to say that his unconscious mind *caused* the lymphoma, but rather, that his unconscious was reacting to the illness in a rather perversely positive fashion. I suggested that during his daily meditation practice, he focus on visualizing a time and place in his life where he felt totally safe and at peace with himself and the world. I encouraged him to use an image from a period well before his diagnosis, but after his childhood traumas, so he could associate a feeling of pleasure and aliveness with health rather than with sickness. (Mind-body pioneer Herbert Benson, M.D., writes about the healing potential of such moments of "remembered well-ness.")

This imagery work helped George to dissociate happiness from disease. His inner healing was also predicated upon freeing himself from the view that "the world is completely hostile, and I'm completely despicable," as he put it. "I've realized that the child in me yearns to be loved but also wants to be strong enough to handle rejection. I've been blaming my parents every day of my life for my unhappiness. Now I can see it's my lack of aware-ness of my essence that's kept me from being happy. Last night, as I was doing the ESSENCE Sound Meditation, I experienced a feel-ing of disappointment that sounded like a long, low moan com-ing from deep in the lower part of my abdomen. Do you think it's a coincidence that that's where my lymphoma started and then recurred?"

George arrived at this perception just before his stem-cell transplant. He responded very well to the treatment, left the hos-pital after ten days, and was back at work in three weeks. Almost five years later, he continues to be fully recovered and healthy. I wonder whether George would have been able to fend off a recur-rence, so common among transplant patients like himself, had he not plumbed the depths of his own psyche with sound and im-agery.

## Treating the Body, Curing the Soul

I am certain that I learn as much or more from my patients about the alchemy of healing as they learn from me. They are all coura-geous men and women whose wish to live helps them to combat, and in many cases to overcome, the illnesses afflicting their bodies.

How they accomplish this remains a mystery to me. As their recoveries progress, I listen carefully to their accounts of what they think is happening. Some are intelligent, others not too bright; some are highly articulate, others tongue-tied. But intellectual acumen and verbal ability don't seem to matter. Those with a brightly burning flame in their souls, regardless of IQ, education, or sophistication, seem more able to arouse the natural self-healing processes in their bodies. Their internal healing systems, with the invaluable help of mainstream medicines, are often strong enough to bring about a complete cure.

I wish I could say that this appreciation struck me all at once in a blinding epiphany. Thoroughly educated in a top American medical school, and equally thoroughly trained at prestigious hospitals, I was open only to what I had been taught to expect. The better I was schooled, the more I had to unlearn. It took me some time to acknowledge that such healing might be possible, and then to observe methodically how patients could awaken these mysterious healing processes in their bodies.

I must add, however, that our concept of healing should never be limited to physical cure. As Michael Lerner, Ph.D., head of the Commonweal Cancer Help Program, has pointed out, *healing* and *curing* are not synonymous. *Cure* refers to complete biological resolution of a disease state, while *healing* refers to a revitalizing and regenerative process that can occur on emotional, spiritual, or physical levels—and sometimes on all three levels in concert. This definition is almost as old as civilization itself. Jeanne Achterberg eloquently describes the shamanistic idea of healing as "an intuitive perception of the universe and all its inhabitants as being of one fabric. . . . Knowing death and life and seeing no difference . . . seeking out all of the experiences of Creation and . . . feeling their texture and multiple meanings." During the Middle Ages, many of the monasteries undertook to practice a compassionate and humanistic form of medicine whose mandate, writes Therese Schroeder-Sheker, was the "care of the body *and* the cure of the soul."

Since that era, and continuing into our own modern time,

most medical practitioners have chosen to ignore the universal truth that healing is far more encompassing than curing; it should be the guidepost and goal not only of the afflicted, but also of those who help them through their struggles. Not only is the healing/curing distinction rooted in important and historic philosophic truths; it can free medical patients from the win/lose mentality foisted on them by many a well-meaning clinician. We mustn't turn the quest for recovery into a sporting event, with the inevitable victors and vanquished—an insidious labeling process that leaves sick people feeling ashamed and inadequate should their illness progress.

If, however, we focus on the broader healing—what Steven Levine refers to as "healing into life and death"—then people coping with illness will not be saddled with so-called New Age guilt. Indeed, the most powerful testimony to healing beyond blame comes from stories of patients who realized a quality of life and capacity for joy they had never before known—at the very times that they intimately confronted their own mortality.

One of these patients was Sheila, who'd been married for several years to Allan when she fell in love with and began an affair with Carl, one of Allan's closest friends. Even after her husband found out about their relationship, he clung to the hope that they might somehow salvage their marriage. They stayed together for three years, until Sheila finally left Allan because she could no longer bear the torment of what she described as "a double life." She and Carl were married shortly after her divorce was finalized.

Two years after that, Sheila received a phone call informing her that Allan had shot and killed himself. She was absolutely shattered; it was as if she herself had pulled the trigger. She started seeing a therapist to deal with her guilt and anguish, but no amount of talking could change what to her was an incontrovertible fact: She was wholly responsible for her ex-husband's death. Carl, too, was distraught. The grief they shared became a deep, wrenching secret that they couldn't escape, no matter how often they visited the cemetery where Allan was buried, no matter how many bouquets of flowers they left on his grave.

I believe that Sheila was almost relieved when she developed pancreatic cancer, perhaps the most difficult type of malignancy to cure. The diagnosis seemed to her a strange form of justice: She'd killed Allan; now it was her turn to die. Sheila flatly refused to attend any of my support group meetings, and she almost seemed to be humoring me when she grudgingly agreed to try a guided imagery/meditation exercise. I don't know which one of us was more astonished by her reaction when the sounds of the bowl reverberated through my office. She wept unashamedly as I instructed her on how to find her life song and led her through a meditation.

Sheila thanked me profusely at the end of her appointment. She said that she felt much lighter and less burdened than she had in longer than she could remember. It was initially difficult for her to harbor any hope of staying alive. Few patients with pancreatic cancer live much longer than one year beyond their diagnosis. The five-year survival rate is 2 to 5 percent. But we continued working together over the next several months as she underwent a treatment course of postsurgical radiation combined with chemotherapy.

I suggested to Sheila that she might also benefit from the Fundamental Sound and Imagery Meditation (see page 153), which unites sound, breath, and imagery to facilitate wellness. The premise of this sound/imagery exercise is that we can develop the ability to manifest in our lives that which we most desire. I believe that while none of us consciously wishes to be ill, or wishes ill upon others, our conscious and unconscious thoughts have extraordinary power to engender the circumstances of our lives— be it disease or health, boundless joy or repetitive misfortune. I also believe that it is our collective birthright to experience infinite love, health, harmony, happiness, and abundance, and that we can develop the ability to manifest those qualities in our lives.

---

### Fundamental Sound and Imagery Meditation

One of the most powerful ways to manifest health and well-being is to conjure an image of your own life force or essence and then animate that image with sound and breath. Begin by closing your eyes and creating a mental picture that represents your essence—a column of pure, vital energy, a rushing waterfall, a bright white light, or any other strong visual manifestation of your essence that feels intuitively meaningful to you. If applicable, invest this image with the power to spur change or regeneration in any part of the body that calls out for healing.

Now further animate this mind-picture by combining it with breath and sound. The power of breath is such because it is the quintessential element of life. *Perceptible* breath is what we feel when the air moves through our nostrils or our mouth. The circular force of breath that draws it in and moves it out is the life energy that comes from our essence. And sound is nothing more than audible breath, a way to manifest our infinite life energy.

The most fundamental sound in every religious practice I know, whether it's Christian Gregorian chants, the Jewish mystical Kabbalistic tradition, Sanskrit, Native American, or Islamic Sufi practice, is the sound *HU*—the basic healing sound that connects all of us with our heart center. This exercise gives you the opportunity to invoke that sound at the same time that you feel the force behind your breath.

1. Breathe in and out through your nose for one minute. Think the sound *HU* as you breathe out.
2. Breathe in and out through your mouth. Chant *"HU"* with each out breath. Continue for one minute.

*(continued on page 154)*

---

(continued from page 153)

3. Breathe in through your mouth and out through your nose. Think
   *HU* as you breathe out. Continue for one minute.
4. Breathe in through your nose and out through your mouth. Chant
   *"HU"* with each out breath for one minute.

As you open your eyes and return to awareness, hold in your mind
the memory of that image, imbued now with the force of sound and
breath. Take it with you as you move through your day, as a reminder
that you were born with the power to bring into your life sustained
periods of serenity, pleasure, and happiness.

Sheila responded particularly well to the Fundamental
Sound and Imagery Meditation, and the shift she was able to
make in her perceptions was nothing short of exceptional.
Through psychotherapy, she'd reached a point where she understood intellectually that she wasn't responsible for Allan's death.
She was still caught, however, in the emotional traps of judgment and blame, and much of her healing depended upon being
able to free herself from the self-imposed iron grip of her guilt.

In time, Sheila came to the emotional and spiritual realization
that it was not her ex-husband she'd betrayed, but rather herself.
That perception enabled her to look at who she was from the
point of view of her essence, and the conditions that had led her to
deceive Allan, so that she could let go of her guilt, and move on.
She lived another four and a half years after her diagnosis, far
longer than most people who have this type of cancer. In some re-
spects, Sheila's story is one of remarkable recovery, given how few
pancreatic cancer patients live longer than even one year.

She died as she'd lived the last years of her life, healed and at
peace with herself. Her husband, Carl, had been able to share in
her healing, and he, too, achieved a sense of resolution during
and after her dying process.

Then there are the stories of patients whose psychospiritual healing coincided with physical cure. The son of a Greek immigrant laborer, Nick was the first person in his family to graduate from college, after which he earned his medical degree, specializing in psychiatry. I met Nick when he was diagnosed with colitis and liked him immediately. After we discussed his treatment options, I asked him why he'd decided to become a doctor. "I almost went blind when I was a kid, and none of the doctors could figure out why," he said. "I finally had to have corneal implants to save my vision. That experience got me interested in medicine, in wanting to help people who couldn't figure out what was going on in their lives."

I was intrigued by Nick's near-blindness. As he proceeded to talk more about his childhood, it occurred to me to ask what psychological stress and trauma might have contributed to his failed eyesight. He told me that his father had been a terrifying and domineering figure who often raised his hand to threaten Nick with a beating. Nick recalled one particular incident when he innocently repeated the "swear words" he'd learned from the children next door. His mother grabbed his hand and thrust it so close to the top of the stove that he felt the heat of the element. "Use those words again," she warned, "and I'll stick your hand right into the fire."

When his father returned home from work, the mother told him what Nick had said. His father raised his fist and shook it in Nick's face, yet another warning of the punishment that awaited him if he used foul language. "His fist was so huge," Nick said, his voice trailing off, as if all these years later the image still had the power to frighten him. "That's the kind of guy he was, always using his macho power to get me to do things I didn't really want to do."

I explored with Nick the possibility that, metaphorically speaking, his blindness had been to some degree an outgrowth of his need not to see the truth about his father or mother. He had spent years denying the full impact of his parents' cruelty, and he had spent as many years denying his own infinitely beautiful and compassionate essence, the part of himself that he'd had to split off, in order to hide it from his parents.

Nick had cured his incipient blindness with transplants, and during his psychiatric training, he'd begun to accept the truth about his father, but hadn't fully integrated the immensely painful and complex feelings he had about their relationship. Both he and I came to believe that his colitis was a somatization of the fear and anger he still held deep within his gut. (The gastrointestinal system, which is packed with receptors for neuropeptides—the so-called chemical carriers of emotion—is notoriously sensitive to emotional states and susceptible to stress-related disorders.)

As with most of my patients, sound meditation and imagery were tailor-made approaches for Nick finally to process these conflicted feelings and transcend them in order to recover his essence. His recognition that he had somatized his childhood pain to the point of actual blindness alerted him to the power of mind in body, enabling him to realize that a similar "conversion" of emotions into symptoms was contributing to his colitis. The sound imagery work—including the Fundamental Sound and Imagery Meditation—empowered Nick to finally let go of his grief and anger, and his colitis gradually resolved itself.

Nick's case is not an isolated one. Many of my patients have used sound, music, imagery, and psychospiritual work to achieve healing that coincides with cure. While cure should not be approached as a foregone conclusion, patients who cultivate a committed willingness to explore the place where individual identity and spiritual essence intersect may find their bodies responding with physical healing. Sound and music modalities now enter the therapeutic repertoire of mind-body-spirit medicine, since they can guide us, laserlike, to the very core of our essence—our highest realization of sound spirit and sound body.

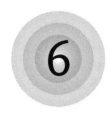

6

# Deep Relaxation and Wholeness

As you might imagine, someone who has just been informed that he or she has cancer and must undergo a course of chemotherapy or radiation to be followed by surgery is likely to experience a rush of emotions, from fear and self-pity to extreme anxiety and anger. It can be hard enough if you've never before meditated to try and sit quietly and follow your breath or focus on a mantra. Consider, then, the challenge presented to a person who's grappling with a newly diagnosed cancer, or any life-threatening disease, for that matter. And recognize that such a diagnosis merely magnifies states of mind—anxiety, sadness, fear of what the future holds—that all of us experience at turning points in our lives.

My experience has been that sound healing techniques usually elicit a state of relative tranquillity in people who are feeling profoundly agitated or apprehensive. The sound of the bowls, other instruments, or toning, used in conjunction with meditation techniques, can calm the mind, soothe emotional turbulence, and induce a psychophysical state of relaxation that liberates us from feeling burdened and overwhelmed. Over time, this temporary liberation becomes a long-lasting freedom from the oppressive bonds of the constricted self.

Sound influences the mental and emotional states, spiritual awareness and experience, and the physical body. While the three are inextricably intertwined, it's possible to peel away and identify the effects of sound on each level. In this chapter I concentrate on the impact of sound on emotional states.

For those of us who are agitated, bowl sounds, vocal toning, singing, and certain forms of music are likely to induce profound states of relaxation. For those of us who have become emotionally frozen due to stressful events or traumas, the same sound interventions may coax painful emotions out of their hiding places in the psyche. For still others of us who are caught in the grip of unyielding sorrow or barely suppressed rage, sound can foster an unexpected equilibrium after a long period of distress.

For Maggie, a bowl-centered meditation practice became a means to cope with a particularly terrifying recurrence of cancer. Maggie had been successfully treated for ocular melanoma, a potentially lethal malignancy, by one of my colleagues, who referred her to me to be her medical oncologist. I ran a series of tests that showed her to be in complete remission, so I told her to come see me again in six months for another checkup. She returned much sooner than that because she was experiencing so much pain in her legs that she could hardly walk. I put her through a second round of tests that turned up bad news: metastatic cancer had developed in her spine and had spread to her liver.

Maggie was devastated when I told her the cancer had recurred. She was in pain, scared and anxious, desperate for reassurance. I understood her fear, but despite conventional interpretations of cancer statistics, I still believed that with the right treatment—and a positive mental attitude—she could begin a healing process on many levels. So even before I outlined her next course of chemotherapy treatment, I told her that I felt hopeful she could learn how to live each day from a perspective of peace and trust. "We hear too much about the people who die," I said, "not enough about the people who live." (She later told me that she'd clung to the words of hope I'd offered her through this one sentence during some of her most difficult, despairing moments.) As part of her recovery, however, she had to find her way to serenity, wholeness, and a deeper connection with her essence.

Maggie had described her life as "immeasurably stressful," and with good reason; not only was this mother of three working part-time as an insurance broker, she was also going to school to get her MBA. She very much needed to create a space in her busy routine for relaxation and self-nurturance. When I suggested that she spend a few minutes each day either meditating or doing a guided visualization, she shook her head, as if to say, *I don't have time for that.* But I must have been so persuasive in my argument that the efficacy of Maggie's chemotherapy would be greatly enhanced by a meditation practice that she finally agreed to let me lead her through a guided imagery exercise while I played one of my crystal bowls.

It took only that one session for her to grasp the benefits of my recommendation. She so enjoyed the experience that she committed herself to listening on a daily basis to the relaxation tapes I'd recorded. She began attending my support group, and soon her husband was coming as well. After her second round of chemotherapy, she gave herself a gift of her own crystal bowl, so that she could reproduce at home the wondrous sounds she heard when I played the bowls at our group meetings.

Three and a half years later, Maggie, whose prognosis with metastatic melanoma to the spine and liver would normally be considered terminal, even with chemotherapy, remains in remission. She works full-time, boasts about her high energy levels, and sees herself as a survivor—someone who's been given "a second chance at life," as she recently put it.

Although chemotherapy surely contributed to her recovery,

Maggie also credits her bowl-centered meditation, which helped her change how she handles tension and pressure. "I really got into it," she told me. "The sound enters your mind and soul, so that every part of you is filled with energy. I visualized the cancer disappearing. At the same time, I used visual imagery to rid myself of the stress in my body, to find peace and harmony, and to find a way to love myself. It was like a cleansing that came over me."

## SOUND AND THE RELAXATION RESPONSE

How and why does sound contribute to emotional wellness and relaxation? Studies and clinical observation suggest that sound interventions elicit the "relaxation response," the term coined by cardiologist Herbert Benson, M.D., for our inborn capacity to counteract the body's fight-or-flight stress response.

When we are under severe or chronic stress, our sympathetic nervous systems go into overdrive, causing the release by our adrenal glands of stress hormones, including adrenaline and the corticosteroids, which have myriad effects on the body.

Our muscles contract as we ready for action, our blood pressure increases, and our breathing and heart rates speed up. Benson, who is now head of the Behavioral Medicine Department and Mind/Body Medical Institute at Harvard University Medical School, conducted pioneering research in the late '60s at Harvard, measuring physiological responses among practitioners of transcendental meditation. He was astonished to discover that—in his own words—"several major physiological systems responded to the simple act of sitting quietly and giving the mind a focus: the metabolism decreased, the heart rate slowed, respiratory rate decreased, and there were distinctive brain waves."

In other words, by practicing meditation we achieve a relaxed state that is the physiologic inverse of fight-or-flight: We become tranquil, and our muscles relax, our breathing and heart rate slows, our blood pressure decreases, and our brain waves take on characteristic patterns of relaxation.

But Benson discovered that meditation was just one among several techniques that people could use to elicit the relaxation response. (He also showed that eliciting the relaxation response not only caused beneficial physical changes, it actually relieved the symptoms of serious physical ailments and helped promote healing.) Virtually any method involving focused awareness and deep breathing, including such disparate practices as yoga, mindfulness, visual imagery, Qi Gong, progressive muscle relaxation, and repetitive prayer, could all produce these same physiologic changes.

Sound must be added to this list. A growing body of evidence and clinical experience now shows us that sound interventions may be used alone, or more commonly, in a synergistic combination with meditation, to induce profound states of relaxation with noticeable—and provable—mental and physiologic dimensions. Music and external sounds (such as the tones produced by Tibetan or crystal bowls) can be combined with our own vocal sounds, and with visual imagery, to radically expand the horizons of the relaxation response as first elaborated by Dr. Benson.

Proof of the stress-reducing power of sound and imagery comes from research by Mark Rider, whose work I discussed in Chapter Five. In one study of twelve shift-working nurses under high levels of stress, Rider tested urine for levels of corticosteroids, hormones secreted by our adrenal glands when our bodies are engaged in the fight-or-flight stress response. He also took body temperatures to assess the degree to which their bodies retained proper circadian (day/night) rhythms—one indicator of body-mind homeostasis. When the nurses listened to tapes of soothing music and practiced relaxation and guided imagery, their rhythms were appropriately balanced and their levels of urinary stress hormones were reduced. On days when the nurses did not listen to the tapes, their rhythms were out of balance and their stress hormone levels were significantly higher.

An enterprising group of Japanese researchers evaluated the effect of music on surgery patients when played immediately before anesthesia was administered. Compared to a control group who did not listen to music, the listeners evidenced significantly higher production of alpha brain waves, indicating states of relaxation, and marked decreases in plasma levels of the stress hormones cortisol, ACTH, and endorphin. By contrast, the control subjects showed *increased* levels of these stress hormones, which are known to diminish the power of our immune systems. This study offers a biochemical explanation for the observation that stress can hamper recovery from surgery, and that music and other relaxation-oriented interventions can, in fact, hasten recovery.

No fewer than nine studies using electroencephalogram measures show that various forms of sound and music slow our brain waves, most notably increasing the amplitude of alpha activity, which is associated with psychological and physical relaxation. (More commonly referred to as an EEG, an electroencephalogram is an instrument that measures the patterns of electrical activity in the brain.) It should come as no surprise, then, that musicians have been shown to exhibit more alpha brain wave activity than nonmusicians. Choice of sound and music is clearly important; several studies have shown that alpha waves increase to the extent that listeners report having "enjoyed" the music. As Mark Rider points out, whether a piece of music or sound is "sedative" or "stimulative" depends more on the relationship between the listener and the music than on the music itself.

These findings support my view that people should choose sounds, sound meditations, music, and imagery with which they resonate. While I believe that the crystal bowls produce sounds with nearly universal appeal, and physiologically relaxing body-mind effects, I also recognize that some people may respond more positively to other instruments—including bells, gongs, drums, or Ting-Sha's—while others may draw maximum benefit simply from the sound of their own voice, as in toning, chanting, or singing. Still others may respond most powerfully to the emotionally soothing or uplifting effects of music, be it classical, New Age, jazz, or rock. I am convinced that each of us has our own perfect, inborn biofeedback monitor that tells us what sounds will have the most salutary influence on our cardiovascular, immune, and nervous systems, not to mention our emotional and spiritual selves.

## SOUND AND EMOTIONAL HEALING

Sound is a uniquely powerful vehicle for emotional healing that works on many different levels: entrainment with emotional states, energetic modulation (since emotions are, according to many theorists, manifestations of biochemical energy), and in the case of music, a highly developed emotional resonance because different types of music evoke such a broad range of emotional states. Given the extent to which sound can influence emotional states and bring about emotional healing for people in distress, I decided to organize an ongoing bimonthly support group for my patients and their families that combines spontaneous sharing and interaction, meditation, imagery, and sound healing, mostly with the crystal bowls.

We generally follow a format similar to the one I use when I meet privately with patients. I begin by inviting people to talk about whatever is going on in their lives, whether it's related to their illness or to any other issue they care to discuss. I've been struck by how often there seems to be an emotional consensus in the room: One night, most of the participants may be preoccupied with the subject of forgiveness; another night, anger or sadness or grief may be the predominant feeling within the group. After everyone who wants to speak has had a chance to do so, I spend a few minutes responding to what I've heard, trying to be attentive to the emotions that have been expressed around the table. Next we move on to the bowls: I ask whoever is interested to lie on the floor, one at a time, on a blanket I've spread, around which I've arranged my Tibetan and crystal bowls. I then spend a few minutes immersing that person in sound vibrations, as described in Chapter Four. The problem I often encounter at this point is that once they've been treated to a "sound bath," people are so relaxed and reflective that they're reluctant to return to their seats and rejoin the group!

I then go on to do a guided meditation, during which I play a crystal bowl and lead the group in chanting the *bija* mantras, or some other combination of other one-syllable words. I start by asking everyone to sit comfortably in their chairs, with hands unclasped in their laps, and eyes closed. After a few seconds of silence, I begin playing a crystal bowl, allowing the sounds to gather intensity before I open the meditation. Opposite you will find an example of a guided meditation with sound, which you can adapt for your own practice, that specifically focuses on the theme of forgiveness.

The meditation techniques I suggest are used by my patients in conjunction with conventional medical methods, *never* in place of them. I've learned we can reasonably expect that opening the doors of the body's self-healing processes will also enhance conventional remedies, that a synergy exists between these healing processes and clinical medical techniques. I've also learned from the families of my patients that healthy people can use sound-based guided imagery and meditation on a regular basis to help them manage the anguish and anxiety caused by the illness of their loved ones.

More and more, I've heard from my patients' husbands and wives, brothers, sisters, or parents, that they were using one or another of the meditation methods I'd introduced to my patients

## Sound and Guided Imagery for
## Forgiveness Meditation

- Take several deep breaths in through your nose, and exhale slowly and quietly through your mouth. With each exhalation, slowly chant the word "HAM" (rhymes with "Mom"). Imagine each breath as a waterfall, flowing into a clear, mountain lake that is located in the upper part of your abdomen. Visualize the lake going deeper and deeper, extending to just below your navel.

- Continue breathing in through your nose, out through your mouth. Now, as you slowly exhale, listen to the sound of the bowl, and chant the word "LAM."

- Imagine yourself breathing in these infinite affirmations: infinite love, infinite peace, infinite harmony, infinite gentleness, infinite kindness, infinite courage. Think about the energy of these infinite affirmations as you take a deep breath in through your nose. As you breathe out, chant the word "LAM."

- Allow the sound to come out easily as you exhale. Don't push it out. Just let it flow from the back of your throat, almost as if you were passively exhaling.

- Imagine yourself breathing in these infinite affirmations: infinite energy, infinite wisdom, infinite grandeur, infinite life, infinite health.

- Take a deep breath in through your nose, and when you exhale, chant the sound "RAM." Now move your awareness to the area around your heart and visualize a crystal ball of white light emanating from your heart. Visualize the source of this white light as being timeless, eternal, infinite, and feel on the deepest level possible that this is your true reality. Understand that all other

(continued on page 166)

(continued from page 165)

manifestations simply appear, and then vanish. Only your essence, which you can find in your heart, is your true reality.

- Examine any chains or walls that you put around your heart to protect yourself from the world, an individual, or a circumstance. Think of a person or a particular circumstance from which you've had to protect yourself at some point, and consider how that need feels in your heart. Feel how it closes down your heart in any way.

- Now, as you chant the sound of "YAM" on a long, slow exhalation, feel the sound moving through your heart like a wave, dissolving any restrictions, any walls, that you've put up to defend yourself. Think about the person or the circumstance from which you've had to protect yourself. But instead of looking at the appearance of that person or the superficialities of that circumstance, delve into the heart of the person or situation. Notice the restrictions that created the situation that has caused you pain.

- Feel your heart embrace that heart, so that your hearts are merged as one. Take a deep breath in and chant the sound "OM." Let the sound remove any restraining walls or chains.

- Send to that person or circumstance energy from your heart— the energy of compassion, the energy of understanding that all beings are seeking to free themselves of suffering. Allow the compassion that comes with that thought to radiate through your heart. Now take a deep breath in, and when you exhale, again chant the word "OM."

- Move your energy back to your own heart, and be conscious of your breathing. Vow to make each breath, each moment, precious and irreplaceable. Realize that the only way you can make

this happen is to remember that moment of being in your perfect harmony, the harmony that comes from realizing your own
essence.

as a way to maintain their well-being and enjoyment of life. They,
in turn, had taught their friends how to meditate, to help them
cope with everything from curing a headache caused by the stress
of getting caught in a traffic jam to sustaining their equilibrium
during a bitterly contested divorce to remaining even-tempered
while juggling a job and three small children.

One man, the chief operating officer of a large manufacturing
company that was in the midst of a bankruptcy reorganization,
told me he'd bought himself a crystal bowl and used it to meditate every day because he was willing to try anything that would
keep him "from flying off the handle" and "drowning in all the
craziness that I have to deal with every day."

Another man I spoke to, a young actor who was appearing
for the first time in an emotionally demanding role on Broadway,
said he felt so drained by the end of each performance that he was
having trouble falling asleep at night. After a close friend who was
a patient of mine had led him in a bowl-centered meditation, he'd
immediately felt so much better that he'd ordered one for himself. Now that he was using the bowl for meditation at least four
days a week, his insomnia had disappeared, and he was feeling
physically stronger, as well. It is quite likely that the actor's use of
sound meditation also helped him stave off the kind of medical
illness that typically develops after long periods of stress and
sleeplessness. I have no doubt that sound meditation is as useful
for disease prevention as it is for treatment.

One young woman, who came to a group support meeting
only because her brother—a patient of mine—urged her to do
so, told me recently that despite her brother's excitement about

the group, she had been very reluctant to attend. She didn't have cancer, so she didn't see the point of traveling for almost three-quarters of an hour at the end of a long workday, "just to sit around and listen to someone play a crystal bowl."

The experience had been not at all what she had imagined. Instead of coming away depressed and disheartened after spending two hours "with a bunch of cancer patients," she said, "I bounced out of the meeting and walked most of the way home, close to three miles. I had come in exhausted by a very difficult work situation, but when I left, I felt totally energized and renewed by the courage and strength in the room. I love going to the beach, and listening to the sounds of that bowl was like taking a dip in an ocean of utterly clear, calm water."

Such reactions are easily understood when we consider how music can provoke an instantaneous change in mood. As babies, our mother's soothing lullabies assuaged our fears and eased our way toward sleep. Research has shown that even in utero, we are aware of and responsive to our mother's heartbeat. Dr. Thomas Verny, author of *The Secret Life of the Unborn Child,* describes studies indicating that fetuses can apparently distinguish between classical and other forms of music; Mozart and Vivaldi were the composers of choice, causing fetal heart rates to stabilize and kicking to lessen, whereas rock music "drove most fetuses to distraction" so that they "kicked violently."

Our innate responsiveness to sound and music is sustained through the stages of development from infancy to adulthood. Many of us have a favorite song that forever recalls—and momentarily re-creates—how we felt the first time we fell in love, danced under the stars, graduated from college, bought our first car, or embarked on another of life's milestones. Hearing a melancholy ballad on the radio, we are suddenly moved to tears, as the melody touches an unconscious memory of a loss never mourned. Conversely, a lively, spirited composition can lift us out of a prolonged mood of despair.

But sound and music are far more than tranquilizers. They can be used therapeutically to help us uncover and resolve repressed emotions associated with past or ongoing traumas. Sound intervention for emotional expression and resolution is a powerful modality that, in my view, can represent a virtual shortcut toward psychological well-being. Put simply, using the bowls, other instruments, or our voices in tandem with meditative practice can help us move through burdensome emotional states far more rapidly than is often possible in standard psychotherapy or counseling. Yet this process does not mean that we sidestep the hard work of transformation.

Consider the case of Barbara, whom I met soon after she'd been diagnosed with ovarian cancer that had spread to many of her lymph nodes. She came to see me because she was pursuing a holistic approach to cancer treatment. Barbara had no family history of cancer, and she was very careful about what she ate. I was aware, however, that she was suffering from a deep sadness that seemed to have nothing to do her cancer. When I asked about her family, her eyes immediately welled up with tears. "My son was born with a severe case of cerebral palsy. He's five now, and doing better than the doctors expected, but it just about kills me that he'll never be a hundred percent OK."

Barbara had asked her oncologist and her surgeon whether her constant state of emotional distress could have contributed to the ovarian cancer. They'd both told her no, absolutely not. She asked me if I thought there could be a connection. "Yes, of course," I said.

I told her that the field of PNI has yielded scores of studies linking distress or depression with a weak or imbalanced immune system, which can be a contributing factor to the unchecked growth of cancer cells. Many doctors are reluctant to talk about this link, because they worry that patients will draw the conclusion that the illness is their fault. I feel exactly the opposite: that developing insight into your life and illness, and the intersections between the two, is an opportunity for growth and healing, not self-blame.

For Barbara, the core issue was her unconscious anguish born of the certainty that her son was not supposed to have had cerebral palsy. She wore her pain like a second skin, and it was all about her son. She believed that fate had dealt him a terribly unfair blow. "How could this have happened to him?" she asked, addressing her question as much to the universe as to me. I couldn't offer any answers that would make sense to her, so I asked instead how she would characterize her relationship with her husband, and how he felt about their marriage.

"He'd probably describe me as 'not there,'" she said. "I'm so involved with taking care of our son that I withdraw from him." When I probed a bit deeper, she admitted that she pushed her friends away as well, that there was a pattern of getting more than she gave, which she'd never looked at before.

Barbara did not seem to understand why she pushed people away, what emotions she was hiding from the world.

But when I asked whether she'd be willing to try to transform these unexpressed emotions into sound and imagery, she nodded a quick yes. The first step was to describe her anguish, which she saw as a gray wall around her heart. I then asked her to give a sound to that image, and after some thought, she replied that what came to mind was a scream of rage. While she didn't feel comfortable about shrieking angrily within the four walls of my office, she was able to give out a growl of angry energy.

I then played a crystal bowl, and she let the sound of her anger merge with the sounds. Here's where crystal bowls can have an almost magical tonic effect; they seem to prompt whatever needs to come to the surface so that, as in Barbara's case, the listener's feelings are validated. Barbara was able to release her anguish in waves of sound. Once it had become safe for her not only fully to allow these emotions into consciousness, but also to vent them, she was able to discuss her deepest emotions with much greater insight.

Barbara said she was angry at God for her troubles and her son's pain. She was also furious with her parents because she wished she had never been born. (I frequently hear similar sentiments expressed by cancer patients.) She withdrew from people because she felt, on some core level, that she did not deserve to live and had little to offer to the world. While the release of her anguish and anger prompted these insights, Barbara still had to do the hard work of transformation.

Her rage was no longer as frightening to her, so I was able to help her transform it through sound interventions. I taught her the ESSENCE Sound Meditation, which I describe in detail in the following pages, and Energetic Re-creation (see next chapter), both ways in which sound mantras are combined with meditation to achieve peace of mind and awareness of essence. She created her own life song, which in effect began to replace the sound of anguish she had carried silently in her heart through the many hardships in her life, most especially the difficulties surrounding her son's illness.

Barbara was going through a process of getting "unstuck," which involves the metaphorical peeling of the onion, getting to deeper and deeper layers of emotion and insight. This is not a magical process with a fairy-tale ending, not a journey in search of a sack of gold coins at the end of the path. Rather, it is a slowly unfolding discovery of self that continues to offer lessons that may be at once disturbing and exhilarating.

Barbara and I continued to work together privately and in the group setting. She also followed my suggestion that she see a therapist, and in time her wellspring of anger dissipated. She underwent a successful bone marrow transplant, enduring all the prolonged stress and pain of such a radical procedure without losing her bearings. She had learned, on an almost cellular level, how her anguish and her defenses against it had limited her relationships. Her husband tells me that Barbara is much more open, and she says she feels better about her marriage and more at peace with the fact of her son's illness. After one group session some weeks ago, I watched her leave the room and was struck by this image: She seemed to be dancing on air.

Barbara's story illustrates how it is possible to "give sound" to negative emotions and start the process of transformation and transcendence. This entire process—which enabled Barbara to reframe her emotional perspective and reclaim her essence—involves seven steps that I call the ESSENCE Sound Meditation. These steps include giving voice to anger and pain, then moving gradually to embrace your essence, a technique that empowers you to move beyond negative emotion into the light of the universal life force.

The Indian text the *Upanishads* states, "Let one therefore keep the mind pure, for what a man thinks, that he becomes." ESSENCE Sound Meditation, and the Energetic Re-creation process, enable us to use sound to keep the mind pure, so that we begin to see the world and live from our essence. In a stepwise manner, we give voice to and validate our pain before surrendering it, and moving toward a wholehearted embrace of our essence, which is infinitely accepting, loving, and capable of healing (see opposite).

The ESSENCE Sound Meditation has healing benefits for people with severe illness, workaday stress, spiritual emergency, or any combination thereof. One such patient was Lindsay, a shy, sensitive librarian in her early thirties who was being treated by another doctor for a soft-tissue sarcoma with postsurgical chemotherapy. Lindsay was referred to me by her oncologist because although she was benefiting from the chemotherapy, the anticipation of it caused her to become nauseated.

The nausea would begin on her way to the hospital for treatment, and it would worsen as soon as she walked into the doctor's waiting room. She would often vomit the minute she came

## ESSENCE Sound Meditation

In the Life Song meditation, you found the sounds that most resonated within you. I have also found that every negative feeling or
emotion has its own sound. Think of a fearful scream (AAH), a sorrowful cry (OOH or EEH), a worried groan (SHHH or UUHH). Before
you begin to do the ESSENCE Sound Meditation, be clear about the
sound of the negative feeling that most disturbs you. Speak it aloud
or scream it as you focus on the negative emotion. The first spontaneous sound you make is the one associated with the essence of this
feeling. You may choose from these disharmonious sounds:

| | |
|---|---|
| SHOO | SHHH |
| AAH | UUHH |
| OOH | DAA |
| EEH | FOO |

Prepare yourself for this meditation by finding a quiet place where
you can sit comfortably with your eyes closed. Take several deep
breaths. Breathe in through your nose, filling the space from your abdomen all the way up to your collarbones with air. Then exhale slowly
through your mouth, reversing the process. Concentrate on each
breath. Observe your breathing for several minutes without trying to
control it. Visualize in your upper abdomen or solar plexus a clear,
still, blue mountain lake. Feel your breath flowing into this lake. With
each breath direct your inner attention to the following positive
thoughts:

**Infinite love, infinite peace, infinite wisdom, infinite harmony,
infinite healing, infinite life, infinite light, infinite success, infinite
possibility, infinite health, infinite hope, infinite energy, infinite
courage, infinite strength.**

Read and familiarize yourself with the following seven steps of the
ESSENCE Sound Meditation. Its purpose is to experience and express negative emotions through sound, then to transcend these

(continued on page 174)

*(continued from page 173)*

feelings by releasing them and reconnecting with your essence, also through sound. This will require a series of emotional and vocal shifts, but with practice they will become smooth and second nature. Once you are comfortable with the seven steps, close your eyes. Start with a few minutes of the breathing exercise, then begin the ESSENCE Sound Meditation.

1. EXPERIENCE Find the place in your body where you experience negative feelings, discomfort, or pain. Feel the exact location and imagine its size, shape, color, and temperature. Visualize this area as pure energy. Pick only one location at a time in your body. Now, experience your negative feelings as one of the above-mentioned sounds. Examples might be AAH (fear), OOH (sorrow), or DAA (yearning). Allow these sounds to vibrate in your throat, opening your mouth to allow the tone to grow. After five or so minutes, gradually shift your awareness to your essence, seeing it in your mind's eye as a white light located above the crown of your head.

2. SENSE Using your life song mantra, sense the harmonic sound of your essence by vocalizing it. Choose mantra sounds from the list on page 125. Examples might be LAM MA SAM or HOME LEE SUME.

3. SURRENDER Release the sound of negative feelings or pain to your essence by visualizing its energy being released upward into the light of your essence. Then, using your voice, revisit the sound of your negative emotion and attach the consonant "M" to the end of it. This is the vocal equivalent of resolution. Examples might be AAHM, RAAHM, or HEEM.

4. EMPOWER Strengthen this harmonious resolution by experiencing your essence as a warm, healing light that you send with each inhalation into the area where you have pain or distress. In-

hale deeply and draw out the sound from step 3 over the course of the entire exhalation. Do this five or six times.

5. NURTURE Nurture the idea of a life free of negative or painful feelings. Sustain the harmony by alternating your essence sound with the transformed negative sound. (Examples: "AAH. AAHM. AAH. AAHM.") Do this for five to ten minutes as you play your bowl or other musical instrument. Try to bring your voice into resonance with the sound of the bowl. As you continue to chant, feel your negative emotions merging harmoniously with your essence.

6. CREATE Create a space for your essence to continue to be your guide by chanting the sound of the transformed negative feelings as you play your bowl. Notice how the sound has lost its disharmonious emotional charge. Continue chanting and playing for two to three minutes.

7. EMBODY Externalize the positive energy by visualizing your entire physical being composed of billions of cells. Visualize the cells as being composed of trillions of molecules, and these molecules in turn composed of trillions of atoms. Visualize the atoms moving, as well as the vast amount of space within and between them.

While playing your bowl or other instrument, inhale through your nose and exhale through your mouth. Recite each of the following infinite affirmations during the entire exhalation: infinite love, infinite light, infinite peace, infinite harmony, infinite trust.

into the treatment room, before any chemotherapy had actually been administered. Her oncologist knew about my use of the bowls and sent Lindsay to me in the hope that sound meditation might help to allay the side effects of the chemotherapy.

I got a graphic and immediate demonstration of the power of Lindsay's fear of chemotherapy when she first came to see me. Although she knew that I wouldn't be administering any drugs, she looked pale when she walked into my office. Perspiration dotted her forehead from the effort of controlling her nausea.

Lindsay's nausea was real. Such "anticipatory nausea" is a fairly common problem among cancer patients, and is a graphic illustration of the mind-body effect: Without receiving even a milligram of toxic chemotherapy, such individuals can experience the same intense nausea and vomiting at the mere expectation of treatment.

Lindsay was so physically and emotionally distressed that she was ready to try any solution I had to offer. I felt that she could greatly benefit from listening to the bowls and doing the ESSENCE Sound Meditation. I started with some simple breathing exercises, then taught her how to play a twelve-inch crystal bowl.

Once she was feeling a bit more relaxed, I asked her to create her Life Song from a list of mantras. I then had her do the first step of ESSENCE Sound Meditation by asking her to *experience* where in her body she most strongly felt the sensation of nausea.

"It's like a tight black band that's choking me around my neck," she said.

When I told her to give that feeling a sound, she responded with "EE."

Next I asked her to find in herself the sound of her essence. After experimenting with several sounds, she came up with "NAM SO HUME."

I asked her to let go of the sound of her nausea by attaching an "M" or "N" to the sound, whereupon she chanted the sound of "EEM" while continuing to play the bowl.

"I already feel calmer," she said.

Next, I asked her to *empower* the release of her anxiety and nausea by chanting "EEM" while inhaling deeply and allowing the sound to be prolonged over the entire out breath. I had her repeat the chant five times.

I then suggested to Lindsay that she *nurture* her newly discovered harmony by alternating her essence sound with that of the transformed sound of her nausea. As she brought her voice in tone with the bowl, she continued to chant "EEM, NAM, SO, HUME" for about five minutes while playing the bowl.

Finally, I had Lindsay *embody* her transformed perspective by chanting her essence sound while visualizing her entire body as trillions of shimmering atoms.

"I feel as if my head is surrounded by a soft, protective mist," she said.

"Imagine you're breathing this energy through every cell in your body," I suggested.

After several minutes, she opened her eyes and smiled at me. "I feel much better now," she said. "The nausea's completely gone."

We agreed that she would use the ESSENCE Sound Meditation before she left home for her next chemotherapy session. If necessary, she would repeat it silently when she arrived in the waiting room. Two days later, she stopped by my office after her appointment. She was thrilled to report that she'd just undergone a chemotherapy treatment without any problems whatsoever, and she was planning to integrate the meditations into her life on a regular basis.

I'm happy to say that Lindsay completed the full course of treatment without any further nausea. The final outcome of her case matched the "reality" she had visualized: The chemotherapy helped check the sarcoma, and she was able to return to work two weeks after her last treatment.

## SOUND AND RITUAL: FROM PERSONAL PRACTICE TO SOCIAL CONNECTEDNESS

As with other mind-body techniques, the healing power of sound is realized not only in private personal practice, but in the broader context of social communities. I started running groups for my patients because I knew that working with sound in unison would create a far greater healing potentiality. Not only does the power of the group apply here, as it does to standard support groups for people dealing with similar issues, but there is something unique about the vibrant blending of voices and tones that translates into a felt experience of unity.

I am inspired by the work of Mark Rider, who has chronicled his use of sound and music interventions for healing workshops he has led in the isolated mountains, deserts, and beaches of North America. As with the ritual uses of sound in shamanic and Native American traditions, Rider encourages participants to use their voices to express their core selves and connect with an essence within and beyond themselves. They begin to emit "noises from a lifetime," that in his view "sweep into a more primitive, phylogenetic consciousness as well . . . flowing freely like some lifeline into the evolution of the universe. . . ."

I was particularly struck by Rider's description, in his book *The Rhythmic Language of Health and Disease,* of how vocal sounds carried his participants into a realm of pure essence:

> Eventually, the cacophony drowns out and gives way to more gentle sighs of relaxation. Slowly, however, more tonal melodies start to emerge. Unfamiliar lullabies begin to rock in the air while others center on a single tone, chanting over and over in a mantra-like style. More and more the vocalizing blends, forming ethereal chords which take on a power greater than that of any single individual's sounds. Like an aural aurora borealis, it hovers there in the air above us, then glides across the room to another location. A second peak is reached, only harmonic this time. People will remark later that this was the point in the choral improvisation that they were "taken out of them-

selves and connected with some energy or power much larger than themselves."

Rider's eloquent description of the personal *and* transpersonal power of sound and voice should be our guidepost. We tend to think of techniques that elicit the relaxation response as antidotes to tension and anxiety, and they are marvelously effective in achieving that goal. However, using sound, meditation, deep breathing, and other relaxation methods solely for stress reduction would be like taking a pleasure cruise and never coming out onto the deck. When we use sound to become entrained with our personal physiologic rhythms—our heartbeat, pulse, brain waves—we also build a bridge that can transport us from a tranquil state to a deeper level of spiritual revitalization, one that links us with the infinite energy and spaciousness of the universe.

7

# Essence and Energetic Re-creation

M ost of my patients are facing life-threatening diseases that could rob them of their most precious hopes and plans for the future. As they look across my desk, I see etched on their faces the evidence of their anguish, not all of which has been caused by the onset of their illness. I see the sadness of their unfulfilled dreams, misplaced guilt, unexpressed anger. I know—both from what they tell me and from what I perceive through their body language and expressions—that they've reached a point in their lives when they've exhausted the familiar coping patterns they adopted in childhood. Mind-body scientist Lydia Temoshok, Ph.D., calls this the "breaking point"— the moment when a person's old psychological defenses begin to collapse. Even those who are most stuck in the past, stubbornly attached to their defense mechanisms, are often desperate enough to look beyond their condition and experiment with a healing modality they might not otherwise have considered trying.

We don't have to be confronted with a life-threatening illness to reach one of life's breaking points, although disease is a common catalyst. A marriage gone bad, a death in the family, financial problems, long-term emotional distress—any of these issues may be enough to prompt us to move beyond our superficial anxieties and concerns.

I believe that we can heal the wounds buried deep within our psyche by contemplating our problems from a broader perspective, distanced from our ego. When we react from a loving, peaceful state of mind and heart, our words, thoughts, actions, and feelings are all connected with the infinite energy of the universal life force. And short of devoting twenty years to studying with a spiritual master, sound is the simplest, most direct route I have discovered to achieve the sense of profound calm that allows us to move into that peaceful inner place, what I call our *essence*.

The concept of sound spirit follows closely on the teaching of sound feelings: Once we move through the shadow states of negative emotion, we can finally transcend our ego-oriented preoccupations. Sound modalities in combination with meditation help us to achieve a spiritual awakening that involves reaching and finally becoming our essence.

Perceiving the world and ourselves from our essence does not mean that we no longer have thoughts, feelings, or personality traits; rather, we are not *defined* by our thoughts, feelings, and traits. Indeed, as transpersonal philosopher Ken Wilber and others have pointed out, we must climb a metaphoric ladder of healing and resolution from one level of consciousness to the next— from "lower" ego-based identifications and body-based emotions to "higher" states of spiritual awareness. Much as we might wish to, we can't skip over all the messy difficulties in our relationships and personal development—the "stuff" we often deal with in psychotherapy, the memories, conflicts, and feelings—and leapfrog our way to spiritual awakening. We have to work through these difficulties, by means of therapy as well as meditation, sound, and imagery. We can then continue with these same methods in order to move to the higher states of consciousness that I characterize as essence. When we find and embrace essence, our personal identity becomes one with a higher identity, and our experience of ourselves and the world is one of boundless compassion and acceptance.

## BEYOND EGO, TOWARD ESSENCE

We all tend to identify the whole of our selves with the limited aspect of mind commonly called "ego." As Ram Dass has written, "Your ego is a set of thoughts that define your universe. It's like a familiar room built of thoughts; you see the universe through its windows. You are secure in it, but to the extent that you are afraid to venture outside, it has become a prison. Your ego has you conned. You believe you need its specific thoughts to survive. The ego controls you through your fear of loss of identity. To give up these thoughts, it seems, would eliminate you, so you cling to them."

It is not as though the parts of ourselves we identify as ego are unimportant or useless. Indeed, the thoughts, feelings, and traits we call *ego* help us to satisfy our desires and remain safe and secure in the world. However, when we identify our complete selves as ego, we make a dangerous mistake, for ego is only a shard of our boundless nature.

My entire approach to healing, including sound interventions, can be summarized as the movement from ego to essence. Our essence can be choiceless, because it is part of the whole of nature; it can be defined as an infinite, loving awareness. Desiderius Erasmus wrote, "It is the chiefest point of happiness that a man is willing to be what he is."

When we identify ourselves as our egos, our blinkered view of ourselves and the world becomes the cause of our suffering; it feeds the isolation, meaninglessness, and ultimate sense of disconnection that leads to despair and, often, to physical illness. When our sights are trained solely on the daily grind of family problems and work pressures, we may realize that we've lost our perspective on the larger reality that connects us with the universe. Our essence, which always exists here and now, seems to slip entirely from the realm of consciousness.

One of my patients buried himself in work as a way to remain dissociated from his essence. Donald's cancer first appeared as a malignant lymphoma, several years after which he developed leukemia. An accountant who was a confirmed workaholic, Donald had taken only one vacation in twenty years, and he deeply resented the time he had to spend away from his office because of his illness. He agreed to do nutritional therapy in conjunction with chemotherapy, but he adamantly refused my suggestions that he try sound-based meditation or any other mind-body techniques that I hoped might help him relax.

Donald was determined to continue working, even after he had to be hospitalized. Although he was running a high fever, he pored over the papers he had spread across the bed until he fell asleep in a chair. I knew from his wife that Donald's unrealistic regimen was totally self-imposed; his boss was an understanding man who would gladly have excused him from his responsibilities. I was therefore sure that he was using his work to avoid dealing with some long-buried wound. But it wasn't until his leukemia worsened and the therapy stopped working that he reached his "breaking point." I sensed that he was finally ready to talk about the pain he carried in his heart, so I asked him, "What happened to you as a child that made you so determined to stay numb?"

Donald's eyes filled with tears as he told me the secret he'd been burdened with for more than fifty years, a secret he hadn't even shared with his wife. "My brother was overseas during the war," he said, "and my father traveled a lot for his job. One afternoon I came home from school and found my mother crying. She said, 'Someone came today from the Army. Your brother's been killed.'

"I was devastated. My big brother was my hero, he meant everything to me. We couldn't get in touch with my father, so for the next couple of days, my mother and I sat by ourselves and cried together. When my father came home, she greeted him with this terrible news. 'Where's the letter?' he asked her. 'There has to be a telegram or some sort of written confirmation.' He made a couple of phone calls and discovered that my brother was very much alive. My mother had made up the whole story.

"What I didn't understand until I was much older was that she'd had a psychotic episode. It was the beginning of her schizophrenia, and eventually she had to be committed to a mental hospital. I was put into foster care because my father was on the road so much, and I hardly ever saw him. All I ever wanted after that was to be like other kids, to live in a house with both my parents. I was so determined to give my wife and kids what had been taken away from me that I tried to create a fairy-tale, Hollywood kind of existence for my family. I figured that if I worked hard enough, I could give them everything they wanted."

In fact, by becoming the absentee father who was always at work, never at home, never available, Donald had unconsciously re-created for his children a situation similar to his own childhood experience. Only now was he prepared to heal that wounded energy by giving voice to his pain. The bowl sounds and ESSENCE Sound Meditation were vehicles that enabled him to remember and express the horrific anguish he had felt throughout his early years. If Donald had solely relied on meditation or talk therapy, I don't believe he would have uncovered this anguish—or the deeper essence that lay below. Sound was the perfect modality to enable him to release himself from what healer Stephen Levine aptly describes as "years of posturing and hiding."

Thus, for the first time in memory, as he was losing his battle with a life-threatening blood cancer, Donald had found his way to his essence. As he continued this work, Donald was finally able to explain to his family why he had separated himself from them; it wasn't for lack of love that he'd missed so many of their early milestones.

There was nothing I could do to save Donald's life. His leukemia was too advanced, and we ran out of therapeutic options. But before he died, he was able to achieve a spiritual healing that allowed him to find peace within himself and with his family.

The Sufis have long recognized that the narrow perspective of the ego is dangerously limited and ultimately misguided. Sufi contemplative and ritual practices encourage people to imagine how God would see their difficulties and their world. How would the center of creation view our problems? We can use imagination, the thinking mind's link to higher centers of consciousness, to find and inhabit a higher perspective—that of essence.

## THE ESSENCE EQUATION:
## UNITY OF CONSCIOUSNESS

When we live from our essence, we can achieve fulfillment on every level of consciousness, from instinctual to intellectual, from emotional to spiritual. No part of our consciousness or being is left out of the essence equation. When we use meditation, sound, and imagery to experience life from our essence, we reestablish our connection with the following:

- **Harmony.** We cultivate harmony when we embrace essence because we recognize that life is to be experienced, not judged, condemned, or repressed. The anxious or repressed mind, fraught with egoistic concerns, can produce only thoughts of the past (regrets, guilt, or charged memories) or of the future (worries, fears, and dreams). When we live our lives solely from these ego-based perspectives, we are no longer grounded in present reality. When we live in self-condemnation, regret, or fantasy, we suppress our life force or essence, which is grounded in the present moment. We reestablish harmony when we use awareness to anchor ourselves in the present, and to allow our life force to flow in an unimpeded fashion.

- **Authenticity.** The truth is not ossified; it is fluid. It is not mystical; it is real. It is not distant, but rather present within each of us. Our true selves—who we are, our essence—is an energy that we can tap into, a felt reality that sound interventions enable us to fully experience. For most of us, the loss of innocence—and authenticity—occurred when we forgot how to *feel* the essence or life force within our own being.

- **Strength.** When you reclaim your essence you come from a position of strength in your work and relationships. You come to realize that your essence is inherently, infinitely strong. I'm not the first to suggest that when you live from a soul level, you gain independence and trust, garnering respect from others because your energy and authenticity are so completely evident.

- **Transformability.** Living from essence empowers you to change aspects of yourself, your health, your environment, or your living conditions that might otherwise seem unalterable. The Sufis say: I am that I become. This implies the possibility of a total break with the past. Who you think you are is just a condition, but you can change the condition. As such, you can wholly transform aspects of your health, relationships, work, beliefs, traits, etc.

Developing harmony, authenticity, strength, and the ability to transform oneself is possible only when you move beyond ego toward essence. But stress management techniques alone are not sufficient to achieve this transition. While meditation has proven to be a marvelous tool for stress reduction, the state of calm and relaxation eventually passes, and we find ourselves once again feeling alienated, uncertain, anxious, or disconnected. We there-fore need to move to an even deeper level, where our perspective shifts from ego to essence. Sound interventions enable us to make this change more surely and rapidly; my patients who practice sound-centered meditations often report an absolute shift in viewpoint to that of their essence. What explains the power of sound in this regard? The simple answer, which I will elaborate shortly, is that our essence is a form of vibratory energy.

One patient who made this shift was Barbara, whose story I told in Chapter Six. Barbara moved through her life with a bro-ken heart, grieving on behalf of her young son who had been born with cerebral palsy. I suggested that during her meditation, she consider the idea that every soul has a particular truth that it's meant to embrace. Through the process of Energetic Re-creation, in combination with the vibrations of the crystal bowl, Barbara began to perceive her son and their relationship from the vantage point of her essence. In the absence of judgment, she was able to replace the ego-based emotions of guilt and helplessness with feelings of compassion, respect, and support for her son's path in life.

## ESSENCE AND ENERGY:
## THE SOUND OF ONENESS

The concept of essence can be cast in psychological, philosophic, transpersonal, or religious terms. But essence can also be understood as energy. The cornerstone of my worldview, which is reflected in many spiritual and nontraditional scientific traditions, is that essence *is* energy. The Japanese call it *ki,* the Chinese call it *chi.* Christianity teaches the eternity and presence of God. Buddhists teach the oneness of consciousness. Lao Tsu called it *Tao.* Wilhelm Reich referred to life energy as *orgone.* Even the Epicureans of Greek times, who generally espoused the belief that we are nothing more than bodies living in a material world, still offered glimpses of a transcendent reality.

I am not the first to call for a science that seeks to characterize the immaterial essence of life, to measure the immeasurable. Unfortunately, mainstream science has largely refrained from showing any interest in the unseen and hard-to-quantify energies in ourselves and our universe. It was Carl Jung who said, "Through scientific understanding, our world has become dehumanized. Man feels himself isolated in the cosmos. He is no longer involved in nature and has lost his emotional participation in natural events, which hitherto has a symbolic meaning for him."

My belief that essence is also energy—a life energy, if you will—explains why I so strongly embrace sound interventions for myself and my patients. Sound is a uniquely potent form of energy medicine that entrains us to the vibrations of our own essence and that of universe.

The whole concept of energy medicine is anathema to Western medicine, yet it has been the foundation of Traditional Chinese Medicine (TCM) for five thousand years. TCM seeks to restore a patient's health by rousing and rebalancing the body's own life force, known as *chi,* which runs in elongated pathways known as meridians throughout the body. *Chi* is believed to enter our bodies through breath, and voice is considered an audible form of breath. We tend to think of TCM as comprised of acupuncture—the placing of needles at specific meridian points to stimulate chi—and Chinese herbs, which also alter and revivify patterns of *chi*. But few realize that Chinese medicine also employs Taoist meditations that involve deep breathing and mantras comprised of "sacred syllables" chanted in deep, low-pitched tones. According to Daniel Reid, an expert in Chinese medicine, "the three most effective syllables are 'om', which stabilizes the body, 'ah,' which harmonizes energy, and 'hum,' which concentrates the spirit."

Thus, the Chinese have recognized that sound and breath are repositories of life energy and can be manipulated in a positive manner to restore balance to our body-mind systems. Once this balance is cultivated, we become centered again in our essence, and the telltale sign is the conspicuous "glow" or "radiance" that we exude.

In my work with medical patients, it has become clear that doctors can use their intuition to empathize with their patients' emotional lives as surely as they can detect imbalances in vital signs or blood lipid levels. An empathetic perspective tells me a great deal about the psychospiritual state of my patient, the extent to which he or she is living from his or her essence. The energy of our essence may be perceived as a fine, harmonious vibration, while ego-based energies—the source of so much suffering and alienation—involves a spectrum of coarser, compressed vibrations. If ego is like a wall around our essence, when we identify exclusively with ego we delimit ourselves energetically and spiritually, denying the luminescent energy of the soul.

Bowl sounds, ESSENCE Sound Meditation, and Energetic Recreation—a voice-based method for dissolving dualities that cut us off from ourselves—entrain us to that fine harmonious vibration that characterizes essence. After sound-centered meditations, our hearts feel lighter, as if the weight of our own egoistic preoccupations has fallen away. Once this occurs, it becomes easier to continue to live and perceive our world from the perspective of essence. How so? When we live in internal disharmony we readily attract disharmony from the world, and there's plenty of that around. But when we live in harmony with the universal energy, we attract people and are drawn to environments that hum with the same positive energies.

We're essentially like stringed instruments: One end of our wires is tuned to the infinite—our essence; the other end is tuned to the finite—the material world, our bodies, our egos. It's not that the infinite is better and the finite is worse. If we are in tune only with the finite, we will be stuck in continual despair, frustration, and disease. If we are in tune only with the infinite, we may lose our ability to effectively negotiate our survival in the real world. Our goal should be to bring the infinite into the finite. Doing so enables us to exist in the present without being imprisoned by our own wounds or egos, or the wounds or egos of others. Bringing the infinite into the finite, we'll never be undone by those who trigger past hurts with their insensitive words or actions. It's our birthright to be tuned to the infinite, and being so frees us from our perceptual prisons of victimhood, depression, obsessiveness, and chronic ill health.

When we utilize singing bowls or practice toning, the fine, harmonious vibration instantly entrains us to the frequency of our own essence. If we are open to the overtones and their resonance, we are reminded in a flash that our authentic selves are indivisible from "something larger"—the higher Self or God, however we define the Absolute. Our egos are tiny little patches of psychological terrain compared with the boundless spaciousness of our essence. The bowls therefore serve as a reminder that all we need to learn in order to heal is already within; sound vibrations are tuning forks that synchronize us to our own true nature.

When we live from our essence we live in harmony—our lives become more like beautiful concertos than the discordant notes produced by garage bands. When we love from our essence, our relationships become positive mirrors. The lovingkindness we project is reflected back at us. In this frame of mind and heart, we intuitively grasp our oneness with the source of all life energy, and we radiate unconditional love to the people we care about most.

I am convinced that life energy, while not yet well characterized in biochemical terms, is both the "stuff" of the soul and the vital force that animates and permeates our cellular structures and higher organ systems. This energy is the root of consciousness, and it is imbued with an intrinsic intelligence. As the French philosopher Pierre Teilhard de Chardin once wrote, "Universal energy must be a thinking energy." We can tune in to the wisdom of the universal life energy through sound meditation.

Sound-oriented meditation alone won't enable us to instantly dissolve all the obstacles in our paths. I have shown how ESSENCE Sound Meditations can be used to move through and transcend negative emotions that keep us stuck in the mud of ego-based concerns. But to move to the level of spirit, deeper explorations and exercises are needed. That is why I developed the sound meditation process I call Energetic Re-creation.

## What is Energetic Re-creation?

Energetic Re-creation involves using the harmony of musical sounds and vocal tones to transcend the conflicts and polarities that exist within ourselves and the world. Most of us are trapped in these polarities, caught between our longed-for connection to the infinite and our obsession with the finite. Put differently, we are by nature dynamic psychic beings, and we often find ourselves going in opposite, or at least several, directions at the same time. One "positive" direction represents the infinite (e.g., "trust") while the other "negative" direction represents the finite (e.g., "fear of the future"). We cannot simply talk ourselves out of the "negative" state and embrace the "positive" one that leads us back to our birthright of infinite love and acceptance. We can, however, use sound to organically—and harmoniously—accept the duality before we transcend it and move on to embrace unity consciousness. Energetic Re-creation is a technique I developed to accomplish this in a systematic fashion.

My patients and people who attend my lectures often ask me, "Why does Energetic Re-creation work?" If you think back to your early childhood, you may recall being taught, as so many of us were, that the world is divided into conflicted states of being: People are either good or bad, rich or poor, healthy or sick, smart or stupid, kind or selfish. When we reconnect with our essence, however, we move beyond this simplistically skewed black-or-white thinking and transcend these states of polarity. Our inner conflicts are transformed through wisdom and love into a condition of harmony, which is the resolution of polarity. When practicing Energetic Re-creation, we learn how to experience conflict (unhappiness, intolerance, or guilt) from the viewpoint of our essence. What results is new insight and a transformed perspective that is truly healing. This applies to every aspect of our emotional states of mind, as well as our relationships, health, and work.

Remember: Our thoughts are incredibly powerful. When we consistently focus on feelings of fear, shame, rage, and sorrow, we manifest these conditions in our lives. By the same token, when we shift our focus to our essence, we bring new levels of healing and homeostasis into our lives.

When we practice Energetic Re-creation, we can achieve

deeper levels of harmony that allow us simply to observe our thoughts as they float through our consciousness. Picture a winter-scene paperweight. Shake it upside down and snowflakes float through the miniature enclosed universe. Trying to solve our problems with the intellectual mind alone is like shaking up the paperweight; we can lose ourselves trying to follow the path of each drifting thought. When we learn how to quiet our thinking processes with Energetic Re-creation, the constant chatter of "monkey mind" finally ceases. In other words, the snowflakes settle and we gain a clear, unobstructed view of our inner landscape and the outer world.

### Energetic Re-creation: The Technique

In our relationship with the world and with others, we tend to react from our ego, whose mission is to defend us from psychological threats. The ego thus views itself as "right," and any entity that opposes it as "wrong." This psychic polarization leads to internal and external conflict. As part of this process, which is fueled by well-intentioned lessons from our parents, teachers, and religious leaders, we "split off" parts of ourselves that society judges unacceptable. Our egos keeps us in line by repressing "unacceptable" sides of ourselves.

Energetic Re-creation allows us to transcend polarity through the discovery of our fundamental inner harmony. The exercise is modeled after the ESSENCE Sound Meditation, since it uses sound and rhythmic alternation, first to express and then to transcend parts of ourselves that we have split off. I have identified five basic states of polarity that most of us experience. Energetic Re-creation does not force us to embrace the positive side of each polarity, but rather enables us to rise above the "negative" aspects of self or emotion by grounding ourselves in our essence. Put differently, we use Energetic Re-creation to give voice to and transcend the five specific polarities that are positive/negative emotional traps from which many of us never escape. These are:

- Trust/Fear of the Future

- Happiness/Discontent

- Love of Self/Lack of Self-Esteem

- Tolerance/Intolerance

- Gratitude/Resistance

Energetic Re-creation follows the ESSENCE Sound Meditation model to allow you to integrate and move beyond these polarities. See the example for Trust/Fear of the Future on page 196. You can follow the same model for each of the five polarities.

## ENERGETIC RE-CREATION IN ACTION

When I think of patients who have taken huge leaps forward along their spiritual path, Bruce immediately comes to mind. A partner in a large New York law firm, Bruce was diagnosed with a particularly aggressive form of lymphoma at the same time that he was going through a bitter divorce. "I guess I didn't exactly have a storybook childhood," Bruce said, when I asked him about his early family life. "My dad was a tough disciplinarian. He beat me up at the slightest excuse, called me all kinds of names, told me I was stupid and a loser."

Bruce had brought to his marriage all the repressed rage he felt for his father. He made his wife the target of his anger, and he treated her as abusively as he himself had been treated. At the onset of his cancer, he and his wife were so estranged that every conversation ended in a vicious fight, and most of their commu-

## Energetic Re-creation Meditation for Releasing Your Fear of the Future and Creating Trust

Prepare yourself for this meditation by finding a quiet place where you can sit comfortably with your eyes closed. Take several deep breaths. Breathe in through your nose, filling the space from your abdomen all the way up to your collarbones with air. Then exhale slowly through your mouth, reversing the process. Concentrate on each breath. Observe your breathing for several minutes without trying to control it. Visualize in your upper abdomen or solar plexus a clear, still, blue mountain lake. Feel your breath flowing into this lake. With each breath direct your inner attention to the following positive thoughts:

**Infinite love, infinite peace, infinite wisdom, infinite harmony, infinite healing, infinite life, infinite light, infinite success, infinite possibility, infinite health, infinite hope, infinite energy, infinite courage, infinite strength.**

1. EXPERIENCE any fear of the future that most concerns you at this time. It may be something that you are afraid will happen at a later date, or a future event over which you fear you have no control. Experience this fear as a sound, e.g., AAH, RAH, or HEE (as in Me). As we move to the next step, shift your awareness to your essence. Visualize it as a white light located above the crown of your head.

2. SENSE the harmonic sound of your essence. Examples might be LAM MA SAM or HOME LEE SUME.

3. SURRENDER or release the sound of your fear of the future by attaching the consonant "M" to the end of it. Examples might be AAHM, RAHM, or HEEM.

4. EMPOWER this harmony by inhaling deeply and pronouncing the sound you created in step 3, drawing it over the course of your entire exhalation. Repeat this five or six times.

5. NURTURE the harmony by alternating your essence sound with the transformed negative sound. Continue chanting as you play your bowl or sound tape for five to ten minutes. Try to bring your voice into resonance with the sound of the bowl. As you chant, feel your fear of the future coming into harmony with your sense of trust.

6. CREATE further trust by chanting the sound of the transformed feeling of your fear of the future while playing the bowl. Notice how the negative feeling has lost its disharmonious emotional charge. Continue doing this for two to three minutes.

7. EMBODY the energy of trust by visualizing your entire physical body as being composed of billions of cells. Visualize the cells as being composed of trillions of molecules, and these molecules in turn composed of trillions of atoms. Visualize the atoms moving, as well as the vast amount of space within and between them.

8. While playing your bowl or other instrument, chant your essence sound and visualize the sound traveling to the space within and between all the atoms that comprise your physical body. Visualize and feel their vibrations becoming more harmonious as you chant the essence sound for two to three minutes. Inhale through your nose and exhale through your mouth, reciting each of the following infinite affirmations during the entire exhalation: **infinite love, infinite light, infinite peace, infinite harmony, infinite trust.**

nication had to be conducted through their respective attorneys. As he described their battles to me, I was reminded of *The War of the Roses,* the Michael Douglas–Kathleen Turner movie about the knockdown, drag-out dissolution of a marriage.

When I met Bruce, his marriage was about to end, his contact with his young son was limited to biweekly visits, and his health was seriously compromised. He had never even considered meditation or any other mind-body technique. But because he was in a state of physical, emotional, and spiritual crisis, he was ready to try any cure I had to offer—and the very first moment he heard me play a crystal bowl, he was hooked. When I subsequently suggested that he experiment with the ESSENCE Sound Meditations and Energetic Re-creation, he plunged into the practice like a deep-sea diver searching for lost treasure.

While undergoing chemotherapy, Bruce attended several of my support group meetings and soon began meditating at home on a daily basis. Through meditation and his practice with the bowls, he came to understand how severely he'd been wounded by his father's physical and verbal abuse. Lack of trust and an inability to tolerate feelings of vulnerability had become a recurring theme in his relationships, whether with his estranged wife, his friends, or his colleagues. As a young child, he'd tremulously anticipated his father's frequent and inevitable assaults. The prospect of imminent disaster constantly hung over him. As an adult, he continued to experience the world as a fearful and uncertain place, where he imagined that at any moment he could be the victim of an unprovoked attack.

During his Energetic Re-creation practice, Bruce gave sound to his fear, after which he alternated this sound with his ESSENCE meditation mantra. In time, this process enabled him to transform his angry, mistrustful feelings for his father and his fear of the future into trusting, compassionate awareness of his own essence.

I had been treating Bruce for about eight months when he came in with a wonderful story that exemplified how his perspective had been altered through his bowl-centered practice and Energetic Re-creation. The previous Friday, he had called his soon-to-be-ex-wife to arrange to pick up his son that afternoon for the weekend. She was coughing as she answered the phone; she told him that she was stuck in bed with a terrible case of the flu, but he should come over as planned to get their son.

On his way to the apartment, Bruce stopped and picked up a bouquet of flowers for his wife. "In the old days," he said, "I would have gone nuts second-guessing myself, wondering why I was bringing her flowers, whether she would misinterpret the gesture, would she think this meant I wanted to get back together with her."

Now, however, he could focus on his wife—who would be spending the weekend alone, in bed, recovering from the flu—from the point of view of his essence. His hostility had been replaced with sympathy, the ability to be open to her pain, a willingness to show his vulnerability as one human being opening his heart to another. He had developed a sense of clarity that enabled him to trust—in the process, in other people, and most importantly in himself.

His rediscovery of his essence provided him with strength and support when I told him that the chemotherapy was no longer working, and his only hope for recovery was a bone marrow transplant. Bruce approached this very arduous process with tremendous courage and grace. Faced with the prospect of spending a month or longer in virtual isolation in order to protect his highly compromised immune system, Bruce decided to take his crystal bowl with him to the hospital.

I will never forget the call I received at the end of Bruce's first week in isolation from the doctor who supervised the transplant. He was doing quite well, my colleague assured me. But it had taken several days for the medical staff on the transplant unit to get used to the strange and wonderful sounds that emanated from his room every morning and evening. I later spoke to Bruce, who laughed as he described the reaction he got when he played his bowl. "At first they thought I was nuts," he said. "But pretty soon, the nurses were stopping by to listen, and then I found out that other patients were coming to sit outside my room so they could hear the sounds, too." I knew Bruce wasn't exaggerating because by the time he left the hospital, five weeks later, I was getting calls from his doctors and nurses who wanted to know where *they* could buy crystal bowls.

Today, Bruce is fully restored to health, and he continues to meditate and practice Energetic Re-creation. Bruce is a very different person from the man I met at his first appointment. He has left the law firm where he worked for many years, because he was no longer willing to tolerate the high levels of stress and the constant traveling that came with the job. He remains in complete remission from cancer—and I believe that one major reason is that he has so thoroughly transformed himself through the use of sound and meditation.

Like Bruce, many of my patients have literally given voice to their profound pain for the first time during singing bowl meditations. They've released the negative energy they'd been carrying from an early age and replaced anger with forgiveness; a fear of their future with a sense of trust in what lies ahead; a lack of self-esteem with a burgeoning love of self. They've come to observe the world from the perspective of essence rather than ego.

People who are ill need to *recognize* the possibility of healing before they can heal themselves. In other words, they need to recognize their spiritual capabilities and power. Too many of us go through life with little or no awareness of the healing energy that lies dormant within. But my patients, more often than not, become their own healers by participating in the world from the vantage point of essence.

When we practice ESSENCE Sound Meditations in order to awaken the soul and incorporate the five spiritual paths of Energetic Re-creation, we establish an equilibrium among mind, body, and spirit. In this state of balance, the mind is at peace, the body is healthy, the spirit soars.

As we move ever closer to a oneness with spirit, to a unity

with the infinite nature of the universe, we are privileged to experience every moment through the eyes of the soul and to realize a life of authenticity. If allowed to unfold without judgment, our life force—our essence—reveals to each of us our unique, divine inner truth and the path we are meant to pursue.

# PART III

# CREATING A NEW PARADIGM FOR HEALING

8

# The Marriage of Intuition and Healing

I was six years old when a heart-sickening thought seized hold of my consciousness: My mother was going to die. Grief-stricken and sobbing, I went running to my parents to be comforted. I don't remember exactly what they said to calm me down, but I do know that my "vision" was not taken seriously. It was chalked up to the typical fears and anxieties about monsters in the closet or snakes under the bed that children often suffer. Then, a year later, my mother began to feel ill. She consulted our doctor and underwent a series of tests. The diagnosis came back: She had cancer.

That horrifying flash of foresight was the first intuitive moment that I can recall experiencing. But the pain of that event—and my mother's death when I was nine years old—made me unconsciously shut down the intuitive part of myself that had been open to seeing beyond the manifest awareness that normally informs our experiences. I had learned my lesson; I didn't want to intuit any more about those who were closest to me. I restricted myself to observing only what was most obvious and apparent—until I entered medical school. There, as a second-year student, I began to learn how to diagnose illness and to note the various physiologic signs of distress.

No one taught me, however, to look beyond the physical manifestations of disease. My patients' body language and facial expressions went unnoticed. Their nonverbal messages went unheard. It was only after I'd practiced medicine for several years, and began delving more deeply into spiritual traditions and practices, that I started to realize the importance of the intuition I'd abandoned in childhood.

When I speak of intuition, I'm referring to the capacity to listen to ourselves and the world through the inner ear of our essence. We are all born with an intuitive sense of the universe, but as happened to me, many of us prefer to ignore that aspect of our consciousness. Rather than respond from our essence and become attuned to the infinite wisdom of the universe, we stay stuck in a fearful, ego-based perspective that binds us to the here and now, with all its inevitable conflicts and contradictions.

My friend and patient, Ödsal, taught me a great many things, but by far the most important lesson was watching him live out the few remaining months of his life. Here was a man who had overcome enormous adversity—exile from his homeland, abject poverty, a wrenching separation from the parents he loved—to become a much-respected scholar with a faculty appointment at a well-known university. He had so much more to accomplish in life, but he'd been struck while still in his mid-thirties with a horrible, debilitating disease that was slowly destroying his body.

Yet Ödsal harbored neither bitterness nor anger nor depression. I never once heard him rail against the Chinese for their barbarous oppression of his country, or lament his difficult childhood, or express any self-pity because he was in pain and dying. Ödsal experienced his reality from the perspective of the universal consciousness, in which there is no place for negative emotions. He approached life—and death—with infinite reserves of love and compassion, gratitude and courage.

Ödsal's extraordinary example became one of my guiding forces as I continued delving into various spiritual traditions. I knew that his unfettered perspective was a lofty goal to set myself. But as I became more immersed in the regular practice of playing my bowls, toning my life song, and meditating, I gradually discovered that I was able to reframe and move past the pain of my mother's early death, which had been the defining moment of my childhood.

Every time I played the bowls, every time I spent half an hour in meditation, my perspective broadened and shifted. Just as the universe is constantly creating itself, I felt myself constantly being re-created, developing greater wisdom and insight into my own issues. I no longer saw the people who came to me for treatment simply as patients who had cancer. Now I wanted to better understand what psychospiritual factors might have contributed to their cancer taking root, what freight they were carrying from their past, what disharmonious tapes they were unknowingly replaying in their unconscious. This understanding, I realized, would come not only from a thorough study of the mind-body literature, but also from developing my creativity and honing my intuition.

## PSYCHIC POPS: ESSENCE AND INTUITION

In her superb book, *Your Sixth Sense,* Belleruth Naparstek describes a phenomenon she often experiences with her psychotherapy clients, something she calls "psychic pops"—moments of "direct knowing and sensing that seem to bypass logic and perception." Naparstek ascribes these moments to "opening my *heart* to this other person, being fully present to them . . . and getting a full sense of them."

Her description reminds me of what frequently occurs between me and my patients. I find that because of my bowl-centered meditations and visualizations, I've been graced with the ability to look past someone's grimace or tears, beyond the expressions of hurt and trauma, and intuit what that person most needs in order to heal on every level. This heightened awareness, which comes from living in my essence, guides me in my personal spiritual odyssey, as well.

Several years ago, I spent a week in Japan, studying with Masayoshi Yamaguchi, the Qi Gong master whose work as a healer has been one of the major influences in my life. Yamaguchi has developed his own form of this ancient Chinese art that involves focusing on one's *chi* or life energy, and learning how to direct that energy throughout the body to enhance health and well-being. As I was saying good-bye to him, I mentioned that I would soon be traveling with my wife and young son to Peru to investigate an herbal treatment commonly used by the natives to fight cancer.

"Must your family go with you?" Yamaguchi asked. "I have a strong sense that you will run into danger there. You will be going to a very isolated area, where there's great poverty. You must remember: The energy from your core is infinitely positive. As long as you are aware of that, nothing negative can harm you."

I appreciated Yamaguchi's concern, but I felt it was unfounded because I'd arranged for reliable guides to accompany us throughout the trip. I thanked him for the warning, and by the time I'd returned to New York, I'd forgotten all about it.

We arrived in Lima on December 23. Colorful Christmas decorations filled every square in the city. After spending the holiday with friends, we left for Cuzco, where we visited Machu Picchu, and from there moved on to Puno. A small town consisting mostly of shanties and dirt roads, Puno is situated at one of the highest points in the Andes, the perfect destination if you wanted to disappear off the face of the earth. When we checked into our hotel about two miles outside of town, the desk clerk told us to make sure we were accompanied by a guide whenever we ventured outside. Unfortunately, our guide never showed up. Yamaguchi's warning began to nag at me, but I brushed it aside when we finally received a call from a man who identified himself as Arturo.

"Nacho is sick," he told me. "I will take you to Lake Titicaca today, then bring you into town tonight."

After a day spent on the lake, where the Indians have lived for centuries on man-made floating islands, Arturo brought us into town and showed us the preparations for the festival of San Blas, Puno's patron saint. We then had a delicious dinner at a restaurant recommended by Arturo for its excellent native dishes, where my three-year-old son happily joined in the music and Andes huaynos dancing.

The evening was getting late when the manager came over to our table. "Arturo had to leave," he said. "He asked me to get you a cab back to the hotel. But don't worry, *señor.* I know all the good drivers."

A light drizzle erupted into a torrential downpour just as we walked outside. There wasn't an empty cab in sight. A fierce-looking man with an unkempt black mustache approached us and offered his service. The manager waved him away. *"No, gracias."* The manager gave him the same response when the man came over to us a second time.

At least ten minutes had passed, and the manager was visibly impatient to get back inside. "I'll send one of my waiters to help you," he said. Moments later, a teenaged boy appeared by our side. The man with the mustache sidled up to him, and they had a brief conversation in rapid-fire Spanish that I could barely follow.

"You can go with this driver," said the waiter. "Otherwise, you may wait a very long time for another taxi."

By now, we were all drenched to the skin, and my son had

fallen asleep in my wife's arms. Both Cathy and I were exhausted after the long day, and we had an equally long itinerary planned for the next day. "Let's go," I said. "The hotel's only two miles from here. We'll be fine with this guy."

I regretted my decision almost immediately, as the driver headed down a deserted road that seemed to go in the opposite direction from our hotel. When I pointed this out to him, speaking both in English and in Spanish, he ignored me and continued driving, his gaze fixed straight ahead on the dark dirt road. Cathy pulled our son closer to her. I could see the fear in her eyes, and I knew this was the moment Yamaguchi had warned me about.

I squeezed her hand to try and reassure her. Then I closed my eyes, inhaled slowly, and on the exhalation began a meditation to visualize myself becoming the energy of my essence. I felt myself moving deeper and deeper toward the core of my being, gathering strength to thwart whatever evil intentions the driver had planned.

"*Sal del carro, ahora!*" he growled at us, as he pulled over to the side of the road. "Get out of the car, now!"

Strange as it may seem, I remained utterly calm as I silently chanted my life song and focused on the affirmations that Yamaguchi had taught me. I visualized waves of positive energy radiating from the infinite essence of the universe, vibrations of the most subtle frequency resonating with the vibrations emanating from my own essence. There was no doubt in my mind that we would be safe.

I opened my eyes and said, firmly but quietly, "We're not getting out. Now take us back to our hotel."

The driver responded by pushing open his door. I don't know who was more astonished when he discovered that he couldn't get out of the car! "*No puedo, no puedo!* I can't, I can't!" he muttered furiously and slammed the door shut.

I could feel Cathy's body stiffen with anxiety as he drove another mile or so along the road, then pulled over again. "*Sal del carro, ahora!"* he repeated his order, somehow managing to make the words sound even more menacing than before.

I refocused myself on entraining my inner sound with the vibrational energies of the universe. "Take us back to the hotel," I said, with a conviction born of total acceptance and serenity.

He pushed his door open again and repeated his attempt to leave the car. *"No puedo,"* he said, almost in a whimper.

The rain was still falling, and the warm air was so heavy with moisture that I felt as if I could almost touch it. Except for the glare of the headlights, we were surrounded by the silence of the black Andean night. The most audible noise was the sound of my sleeping son's quietly rhythmic breathing. The driver turned and scowled at me over his shoulder. I met his gaze and continued to visualize the link between the universe and my life force.

After several moments, he turned back around, executed a hasty U-turn in the middle of the road, and drove us directly to our hotel. He was still mumbling to himself as he sped away in a cloud of dust.

I'm pleased to report that the rest of our trip to Peru was far less eventful. As to why the driver couldn't get out of the car, to this day I have no simple or clear-cut explanation. Perhaps his guilty conscience prevented him from carrying out whatever he'd planned to do to us. But this particular episode is one I will never forget—and not simply because of the drama of the situation. It represents for me not only a stunning example of the power of intuition, but also the truth of Yamaguchi's counsel that our infinitely positive and loving essence is the most potent weapon we have for battling aggression and negativity.

The Japanese word for "intuition" is composed of three characters that represent these three concepts: direct, perception, and power. When this linguistic fact was first pointed out to me, I couldn't help but marvel at the compact elegance of this paradigm for delving into the nature of intuition. Simply put, intuition refers to our "power to perceive something directly," according to Masami Saionji, the chairperson of the World Peace Prayer Society, whose thinking has greatly influenced both my teacher, Yamaguchi, and myself.

"The word 'intuition' refers to the functioning of an unseen power originating at the source of our life," writes Saionji. "Developing your intuition means cultivating your faculty for allowing the vibrations from heaven to be received directly into your body."

Imagine, if you will, being able to dip into your well of intuitive power as you struggle to overcome a serious illness or challenging life crisis. I have worked to cultivate this capacity in my patients, not through mystification or the power of magical thinking, but by systematically helping them develop their innate sense of intuition with sound, meditation, and imagery. (Seemingly supernatural occurrences, such as the one I report above, can and do happen. But I do not suggest to patients that they can wish or meditate away their cancers or other diseases. Rather, I emphasize that entraining themselves with universal energies and following their deepest instincts is a sure path to healing, if not physical cure.)

Moreover, the human capacity for intuition and its effects on the body, on relationships, and on one's environment is not grounded in the occult or esoterica, but rather in hard scientific investigation by some of the great minds of physics and philosophy.

## AN OCEAN OF ENERGY: NONLOCAL CONSCIOUSNESS

Mind-body scientists believe that meditation, guided imagery and visualizations, prayer, and Qi Gong are "right brain activities," because the right hemisphere of the brain is the seat of intuitive, emotional, and creative impulses and processes. Such activities are thought to promote our ability to retrieve images and information stored in the unconscious, which in turn enhances our capacity for accessing the universal wisdom that we often refer to as intuition. It is when we sit in silent meditation, or practice the meditative exercises known as Qi Gong, or attune ourselves to the finer vibrations of the universe while playing our bowls, that our brain waves patterns shift. We move from the actively engaged state of beta, through alpha—a more neutral, inwardly focused state that's commonly achieved simply by shutting our eyes, into theta, a frequency range on the border between sleep and wakefulness that's associated with profound levels of relaxation.

Elmer Green, Ph.D., spent many years at the Menninger Foundation, researching biofeedback, and other means of self-regulating physiologic functions. In the early '70s, Green and his wife and collaborator, Alyce, undertook to investigate the specific properties of the theta state. An earlier Japanese study, which had examined how meditation affected brain wave patterns among Zen Buddhist priests and their disciples, reported that as the subjects entered more deeply into a meditative state, alpha levels decreased and theta wave predominated.

In their own research, the Greens and their colleagues discovered that through biofeedback instruction they could teach people how to control their shifts from beta to alpha and theta states. Moreover, almost half of the subjects reported a high incidence of ESP episodes, especially while they were in theta. "We found theta to be associated with a deeply internalized state," Green wrote in *Beyond Biofeedback.* "The state of deep quietness of body, emotions, and mind . . . achieved in theta training seems to build a bridge between conscious and unconscious processes and allows usually 'unheard' things to come to consciousness." Indeed, says Belleruth Naparstek, such highly respected and long-time intuitives as Rosalyn Bruyere, Emilie Conrad-Da'oud, and Ken Cohen have been found to spend many of their waking hours in theta state.

The theta brain wave studies tell us that there is a level of human consciousness in which we are more highly attuned to inner realities as well as to "other realities" outside ourselves—beyond the border of skin that defines the "local" self. But scientists are moving to far more encompassing explanations of what physician Larry Dossey calls "nonlocal consciousness." We are learning that our minds, indeed our personal selves, may be indivisible from the greater consciousness of the universe, or to put it more spiritually, the essence or absolute. In the vanguard of this understanding is a small group of theoretical physicists whose work is shedding light on the nonlocal nature of human awareness. We are learning that prayer, visualization, sound, and intuition are processes that help us move our minds beyond conventional borders of selfhood, enabling us to draw from a truly infinite consciousness.

The late David Bohm was in the forefront of physicists who propounded this theory of nonlocal consciousness. Bohm believed that the universe is a vast ocean of energy, that our constructs of time are illusory (we exist in a sequence of present moments; past and present are basically meaningless); that the objective world as we know it, which he referred to as the "explicate order," is actually infused with and animated by the ocean of energy, or implicate order; and that these two realms are part of an enormous, flowing whole he referred to as the *holomovement*. Belleruth Naparstek sums up Bohm's vision thusly:

> We actually inhabit a universe where every point is interpenetrated by every other point. This universe is made up of the implicate order, a vast ocean of living, conscious, intelligent energy underlying, surrounding, overlaying, and interpenetrating the ordinary world of our experience. And embedded in this implicate order is the superimplicate order, a vast—in fact, infinite—information field, a protointelligence organizing and directing the energy of the

implicate order and enfolded within it. From the implicate and superimplicate orders (of which there are an infinite number in an infinite array or spectrum) is derived the manifest world of our experience.

From this vantage point, human consciousness may comprehend aspects of the implicate and superimplicate orders that extend far beyond the seeming surfaces of reality. Naparstek captures Bohm's notion of nonlocality: "Because everything is enfolded within everything else, this vast information field is everywhere, inside of us and outside of us. It coexists with and pulses in our ordinary reality. Because of its qualities of nonlocality, information from all time is co-present and available in its entirety."

Human intuition, then, can be thought of not merely as a property of the brain or psyche, but as an ability to tap into the implicate and superimplicate orders. Why is sound such a powerful modality, enabling us to swim in this vast ocean of energy? In summarizing one of Bohm's beliefs, Naparstek strikes to the heart of the matter: "Similar things pulsate in a similar way and instantaneously communicate with and influence one another at these subtle levels through a kind of synchronized resonation."

I couldn't imagine a better definition of entrainment, the synchronous influence of one energy system on another. And as I have documented throughout this book, the sound of music, overtones, singing bowls, and other sacred instruments can indeed influence mind and body "through a kind of synchronized resonation." This also suggests that sound modalities can fine-tune, or even bring forth for the first time, our native intuition—our grasp of the implicate order that fills and surrounds us. What Bohm calls "the implicate order" I call "essence," but the terms matter less than whether we commit ourselves to practices that open our minds and hearts to the "something greater than ourselves" into which our individual selves are embedded.

While Bohm's theories offer a relatively complete and profound understanding of the implicate order, theoretician and researcher Itzhak Bentov gave us a more concrete scientific understanding of how we can be informed by this boundless universal energy. In his book *Stalking the Wild Pendulum,* Bentov described a theory of solid matter as nothing but pure vibration, characterizing particles as "wave packets." The human body is therefore also composed of vibrations, oscillating at a rate of approximately seven times per second; however, we can't generally perceive these quick and subtle movements in our normal waking states.

The oscillations of Bentov's wave packets, and everything else in the universe, for that matter, behave like a pendulum: A still point is reached each time the pendulum has moved as far as it can in one direction before it begins to move in the opposite direction. According to Bentov, all oscillating systems have this property. Naparstek captures the relevance of Bentov's idea to human intuition:

> Our body is the pendulum. It oscillates up and down at a rate of about seven cycles per second and therefore reaches a state of rest at the rate of fourteen times a second. This means that fourteen times every second (and probably a lot more, but at least that), we are expanding at a very high speed through subjective time into objective space. In no time at all, we come back again, but during that "no time" we have been out into other dimensions and realities, dispensing and collecting information. . . .
>
> Sometimes, under certain circumstances, we are capable of bringing the data back into our three-dimensional world—if we're wired sensitively or if we've trained our minds to do so. Both Bohm and Bentov felt that meditation was the best way to train the mind to spend longer periods of subjective time out there in space-time during those blinks away. This is because meditation lowers the frequen-

cies of our brain waves and, in so doing, expands the perceived time that we are "out."

Bentov's pendulum concept helps us to understand that we can "swing" toward those points of stillness, during which we can "dispense and collect information" from other dimensions—the implicate and superimplicate orders, to return to Bohm's concepts. In my experience, sound entrainment and deep meditation are practical and powerful tools to enable us to make the most of these little pauses in the time-space continuum. The "information" we gather and dispense can help us to understand ourselves and others, discover what we need to heal our bodies, and realize our deepest spiritual nature.

## INTUITION AND THE WISDOM OF THE BODY

Sound healing practices have helped me to develop my own intuitive sense, and the resulting insights I've had into emotions and feelings have greatly benefited my patients. I never rely on intuition to make decisions about medical treatment, nor do I consider myself a psychic or "medical intuitive." But I can recall more than a few instances when I've become aware of an emotional or spiritual concern that might hinder my patient's well-being, and I've been able to use that awareness to help that person overcome previously unacknowledged blockages to healing.

One such patient was Wendy, who had discovered a lump in her breast three months before she finally decided to see a doctor about it. The delay had severe consequences. By the time she was diagnosed with breast cancer, the tumor was huge and her lymph nodes were found to contain metastatic disease. Wendy would require far more aggressive chemotherapy to try to stave off the now substantial risk of a recurrence.

After we talked about her treatment, I asked her why she'd

waited so long before coming in for an examination. Wendy's shoulders sagged in resignation. "I thought maybe it was a cyst," she said. "I kept hoping it would just go away."

There was another reason she'd put off going to see her doctor. She'd recently left her job and lost her medical insurance. She didn't have enough money to cover the treatments, but she was planning to apply for Medicaid. I asked her how she'd paid for the surgery.

"I have a friend who owns her own business and is very wealthy. She insisted on putting out the money for the operation." Wendy glanced at me quickly, almost as if she expected me to show some sign of disapproval. Then she said, "She wants to pay for the chemo, but I feel awful about letting her do that. And of course I'm going to pay back whatever she's already spent on me."

She lowered her head and kept her gaze averted. The message that came to me then was that here was a person who felt utterly unlovable. Her energy seemed sluggish and blocked by a shame that had festered inside her for many years.

My intuitive hunch was that she'd felt unloved since childhood, that she'd been failed by one or both of her parents. I also sensed that she'd never dealt with this issue, so I gently encouraged her to tell me about her family.

She was the third of five children, she said. Both her parents had been alcoholics for as long as she could remember. They'd moved around frequently because her father couldn't keep a job, and there often wasn't enough money to pay the rent.

She'd had a series of tumultuous romantic relationships and gotten married at twenty-five to a man who was, not surprisingly, an alcoholic. He'd walked out on her three years later, but not before racking up a pile of debt on her credit card and cleaning out what little money there was in their joint checking account. "I wanted kids," she said sadly. "I guess it's a good thing he didn't let me have any."

"Why do you think it's so terrible to let your friend pay for your treatment?" I asked.

"I don't know," she said.

"Why do you think she wants to give you the money?"

She shook her head. She didn't have an answer for that, either.

"Maybe it's purely out of love," I suggested.

Wendy burst into tears.

"This is hard for you because you feel so unlovable," I said. "You can't accept anything—even if it could save your life—because you feel you don't deserve it."

She stared at me in astonishment. It didn't require great intuition to know what she was thinking; how did I know what she was feeling? Because in that moment, I had myself experienced the heaviness that lay on her heart. The image that came into my awareness was that of a heavy boot holding her down, preventing her from accepting love, from letting anyone get close to her.

With any luck, chemotherapy would decrease her chances of a recurrent cancer. But no amount of chemicals could destroy the disease of self-loathing that was killing her soul. As a doctor, I could treat only the cancer. As a healer, I could intuitively help her reconnect with her essence by sharing with her whatever wisdom the universe had chosen to impart to me.

## SACRED SOUNDS AND PICTURES: DEVELOPING THE INTUITIVE MIND

As a small child, Jill Purce was visiting an isolated island off the west coast of Ireland with her parents. "The only other people in the small boat were the old women of the island returning home," says Purce. "A violent storm blew up and it seemed obvious to all of us we were going to drown. Suddenly the women began to sing with an ancient power and deep passion. Almost at once our fear dissolved, waves of strength surged into us, until finally we were overcome with feelings of bliss and enchantment."

Purce, the author of *The Mystic Spiral* and a renowned authority on the subject of sacred chanting, remembers this incident as her "first transmission of the power of the voice." Since then, she has spent many years studying ancient vocal techniques and the power of group chanting. "My aim is not modest," she says. "I am trying to re-enchant the world, which means to make it magical through chanting."

She intends to accomplish her goal by leading workshops in her native England, the rest of Europe, and America, focusing on the therapeutic use of sound. Purce, who studied overtoning with the Tibetan Chantmaster of the Gyuto Tantric College, is particularly taken with Mongolian overtone chanting, which "involves a single note only, but by modulating all the resonant cavities including the shape of the mouth, you make audible, high, bell-like sounds which float above the continuous bass note in a way which makes people think of the music of the spheres. The overtones are the component parts of the fundamental note being chanted, and are normally too quiet to be audible. Here they are filtered in such a way that they can be heard louder than the note itself."

Purce's definition is as good an explanation as I've ever heard of overtoning, which I discussed in Chapter One. Purce believes, as I do, that the breath is a bridge between our voices and our minds, and that "through working with the voice we can learn to enter the state the Tibetans know as 'rigpa,' the awareness which combines emptiness with clarity." It is while we inhabit that state of awareness—particularly when we use our voices in concert with singing bowls—that we entrain with the rhythms of the universe and restore harmony to mind and body on cellular levels that may even affect our DNA.

As I've mentioned repeatedly, the combination of visualization and sound healing methods can engage layers of imagination and intuition that further extend psychospiritual and physiologic healing processes. The foremost practitioner of sound/image modalities is Helen Bonny, Ph.D., a music therapist who developed the Guided Imagery and Music (GIM) technique, which draws on carefully chosen pieces of classical music to summon from the subconscious deeply embedded images and mythic representations.

GIM evolved out of research conducted by Bonny and others during the 1960s at the Maryland Psychiatric Research Center; the studies were designed to explore human consciousness through a combination of hallucinogenic drugs, including LSD, and more traditional forms of psychotherapy. Bonny eventually concluded that drugs were unnecessary, because classical music provided a very effective road map for delving into the deepest strata of the human psyche and facilitating an emotional catharsis. Drawing upon Jung's use of mythic symbols to steer us to the unconscious, she created a music- and image-oriented method in which a healing partnership is established between the client or "traveler" and GIM-trained "guide." The client is encouraged to enter into a state of deep relaxation while listening to tapes of preselected programs of classical music, depending on what type of feelings the guide hopes to evoke and what issues the client wants to work on. As the music—which becomes, in a sense, the "cotherapist"—unfolds, a rich stew of symbols, images, and fantasies rises to the surface of consciousness, there to be jointly explored by the client and the guide.

Sara Jane Stokes, Ph.D., codirector of the Mid-Atlantic GIM Training Institute, recounts a moving example of the power of GIM in the story of Doris, a client in her mid-forties, who had been grappling with personal and professional identity problems. In one particular session, Stokes chose to play the "Positive Affect" tape, which includes the Adagio for Strings and the Offertory and Sanctus from *St. Cecilia Mass* by Gounod. Doris, who strongly identified with the musical themes of union and rebirth, described a symbolically fertile and triumphant image that represented a jubilant sense of wholeness.

"As the music held me in its power and strength," she wrote afterward, "I had the feeling of warm afterbirth pouring out of me, and a penetrating light and euphony of a full-bodied major chord played by a full orchestra surrounding me. When the delivery was over, I discovered I had given birth not to a child, but to myself—a huge brilliant sunmoon. I was alive with ecstasy!"

Among the hallmarks of GIM is that the imagery is spontaneously evoked, without any specific instructions or directed goals. The clients become, in a sense, their own healers; both they and their guides must trust and rely on their intuitive capacity to interpret the symbols and images that arise throughout the session. Similar in spirit to the healing work I do with my patients, the ultimate objective of GIM is to provide a safe emotional space in which the clients can heal their wounded psyches by listening to and honoring the infinite intelligence of the universe. Carol Bush, a licensed GIM guide and author of *Healing Imagery and Music,* reminds us that Ken Wilber "has said that human beings are multi-layered manifestations of universal mind. In GIM the music becomes a superb catalyst for an experience of this universal consciousness."

Bush suggests the exercise opposite, which you can do by yourself to explore a self-directed version of the GIM technique.

Albert Einstein, unquestionably one of the greatest minds of the twentieth century, had this to say on the subject of intuition: "The intellect has little to do on the road to discovery. There comes a leap in consciousness, call it intuition or what you will, and the solution comes to you, and you don't know how or why."

That "leap in consciousness," which I frequently experience when I meet with patients, has helped me as a healer-physician to diagnose ailments of the mind and spirit, as well as the body. It has also helped me to become more fulfilled and creative in my work and personal relationships. Psychologist Lawrence LeShan,

## Exercise

Find a quiet place where you can relax for fifteen to thirty minutes without interruption. Have a CD or cassette player within reach, and a notebook or journal.

- *Formulate a Focus*  Identify an area of concern, or one for which you wish to generate a flow of creative ideas. Write it in your journal. This step is like posting a question to your inner self. In order for your focus to be productive, it is necessary to have a sense of personal relatedness to the issue. Write down any random thoughts that are on the surface of your mind, as if you were "clearing the decks" before beginning a journey. Write a brief statement in your journal. Then choose the music that fits.

- *Choosing the Music*  **Earth Music** provides a "safe container" with music that is supportive while stimulating a wide range of imagery experience. It invites you into the reveries and feelings of the inner world.

    Beethoven: Symphony no. 7, movement II

    Beethoven: Symphony no. 9 in D Minor, movement III

    Brahms: Symphony no. 4, movement II

    Debussy: *Prélude à l'après-midi d'un faune*

    Ravel: *Daphnis et Chloé,* suite no. 2, part 1

**Fire Music** evokes strong feelings that encourage exploration of the more "heated" emotions. This music provides the intensity that strong feelings require in order to be expressed.

    Bach: Toccata and Fugue in D Minor

    Brahms: Piano Concerto no. 2, Allegro non troppo

    Brahms: Symphony no. 3 in F Major, op. 90, movement I

    Debussy: *La Mer,* movement I

**Air Music** releases the imaginative forces. While stimulating a free flow of creative connections, it awakens the creative imagination.

(continued on page 224)

*(continued from page 223)*

The fluidity and wide sweep of the sounds helps to evoke multiple impressions for creative brainstorming.

Bach: Orchestral Suite no. 3 in D Major, movement II

Beethoven: Symphony no. 9, movement I

Berlioz: *Symphonie fantastique,* movement II

Ravel: Introduction and Allegro

**Water Music** is emotional music. It awakens and allows feelings to come to the surface to be explored and, within the imagery, to be expressed. Water music is especially evocative of more tender emotions.

Bartók: *Music for Strings, Percussion, and Celesta,* movement I

Beethoven: String Quartet in C Major, op. 131

Brahms: Symphony no. 2, movement III, Andante

Debussy: *Dances Sacred and Profane*

- *Relaxation Exercise* In order to change to an inward focus, the body requires a brief interval to relax. This interval provides a signal to the body-mind that enables it to change gears, as it were, and attend to the images and sensations that will soon appear. Loosen any constricting clothing. Close your eyes and begin to breathe deeply, turning the focus inward while scanning the body for tension spots. Allow yourself to feel, with every outflow of breath, that you are releasing tension. Feel the muscles relaxing. Allow your shoulders to release, your neck and head and any other places where you are holding tension. As you breathe out tension, you will actually be eliminating tension and stress. Beginning with your feet, progressively focus your breathing on your lower body, then midsection, shoulders, and head as you continue to consciously breathe out tension from the whole body.

- *Traveling in Inner Space with Music* As the music begins, surrender to it. Allow it to carry you into an experience. Keep the attention focused on the emerging imagery. As a scene forms, let yourself become involved with it. If, for example, a forest scene emerges, enter it. If a path is seen, follow it. If a person appears, you can talk with him or her. Since the intuition is often an active force in this process, allow yourself to sense what to do or where to go with the imagery. Whether you are fully aware or not, the music carries the imagery along, encouraging it to take on dimension, movement, feeling, and drama. Be spontaneous and let the music take you to . . . wherever you need to go!

- *Returning*  As the music ends, spend a moment reviewing what you have experienced. Allow yourself to return to your normal state gradually. The images and impressions are still in raw form, somewhat like recalling a dream. They may require associational processing to make connections to your original focus. To begin this postsession work, write down what you remember along with any associations that immediately occur. Give the experience a title. This helps to organize large amounts of associational material. It works best to give a title that relates to its content rather than one that is allegorical.

- *Write a Brief Account of the Experience.*

**Bon voyage!**

Ph.D., well known for his pioneering psychotherapeutic work with cancer patients, has spoken metaphorically of how we all need "our own song to sing" so that we can each find our own unique way of "being, relating, and creating."

When we sing our life songs and practice Energetic Re-creation in harmony with the sound of the bowls, we begin to listen to the sounds and memories that are stored within our bodies, to experience the feelings of hurt that we've long repressed. We move into a different realm of consciousness, one in which our perspective shifts from the limited awareness of the here and now to an infinite appreciation of the universe.

From that infinite perspective, we can start to identify ourselves as who we are in the process of becoming, rather than who we have been. With that in mind, I share with you this simple, meditative reflection by Masami Saionji on the subject of intuition:

> *Intuition always exists in you.*
> *It was there from the beginning.*
> *It is not man-made, nor does it need to be.*
> *It is within you.*
> *It is around you.*
> *It is you.*
>
> *There is no need to search for it.*
> *You simply need to become aware of it.*
> *Become aware that you are a spirit from God.*
>
> *You are no longer asleep.*
> *You are no longer dreaming.*
> *You have come to see the truth.*
>
> *The truth is*
> *That you are a child of God,*
> *Shining brightly.*

## 9

SOUND SYNTHESIS:

# A New Paradigm for Holistic Medicine

In his illuminating book *Recovering the Soul,* Larry Dossey, M.D., describes what he calls "Era III medicine," a time when "minds are . . . omnipresent, infinite, and immortal. . . ." Dossey's concept moves us beyond a definition of medicine that is based on methods such as chemotherapy and surgery that treat only the body, or on the even more wide-ranging model of mind-body therapies. Era III medicine relies on the healing potential of nonlocal consciousness, says Dossey, whose understanding of our transcendent states of awareness reflects the concept of essence, as I've defined it throughout this book. Dossey believes that consciousness can be nonlocal because, "like the Divine, it is infinite in space and time and is ultimately One."

Dossey's notion of an infinite consciousness dovetails perfectly with the principles and practices of sound healing. When I sit with patients, either individually or in a group, and we share the resonant sound of the crystal bowls, merged with our own voices, the space around us is filled with vibration. We are thus reminded that we are all connected by a universal energy, and that consciousness is indeed "infinite in space and time."

Sound in its myriad guises can be used to traverse what Ken Wilber calls the "spectrum of consciousness"—the bands of awareness that range from the sensory and physical through the emotional and cognitive to the ultimate or transcendent. As noted, Wilber says that we must fully embrace each level, and then move higher—as if ascending the rungs of a ladder. Sound and voice literally resonate on all of these levels, helping us to fully integrate them, and to move toward that ultimate awareness—a direct experience of the infinite.

Whether we suffer from physical illness or are blessed with good health, we all yearn for wholeness and spiritual connectedness. Sometimes, however, that yearning is obscured by our own emotional blocks, as it was from an internal medicine patient of mine, a fifty-nine-year-old former actress. An alcoholic who had never accepted her many successes on Broadway, Evelyn walked through life feeling hopeless and despairing. In the years since she had retired from the stage, her drinking had gotten worse. She came to see me on this particular occasion because she had been coughing for days and was having chest pains. Her large brown eyes, usually so expressive, were dulled by the combined effects of fever and too many bottles of Scotch.

She seemed to be teetering at the precipice of a physical and spiritual crisis. I was deeply concerned about her physical condition, which turned out to be a serious case of pneumonia. But I felt I also had to address head-on the issues behind her drinking.

Although I knew she wouldn't have an answer, I asked her why she was drinking again.

Her response was exactly what I'd expected. "I don't know. Sometimes I just go on binges." But then she surprised me. "I know I'm really hurting myself. I wish I could stop."

"What feelings are you trying to numb?" I asked, getting straight to the point.

She shrugged. "Just life, I guess."

I'd known Evelyn for quite a few years, and I was very fond of her. Her answer deeply saddened me, but perhaps because my heart was open to her in that moment, I had one of my intuitive flashes. I could almost reach over and feel the crushing burden of anguish that had weighed her down since childhood. Yet in all the times I'd seen her, she'd never given any hint of having had a particularly difficult past. Nevertheless, I now knew that something terrible had happened to her as a child.

"I have a sense that you suffered deeply when you were a little girl," I said bluntly. "Do you remember any negative incidents or traumas?"

Even today, Evelyn is a marvelous actress, but this was one time she couldn't mask her shock. "I haven't talked about this since I was seventeen. I haven't even thought about it," she said, as she began to weep. "It won't do any good now. I'll never be able to deal with it. My life is already ruined and over."

"You can release it right now," I said. "You can be rid of your secret by the time you walk out of here."

She stared at me, silently challenging me to make good on my promise. But I could also see a change in her expression, as if the mere fact that someone was willing to listen was enough to produce a shift in her energy. And then the words came tumbling out of her, so quickly that I realized she'd kept them pent up for a very long time.

She'd grown up in a small town in Pennsylvania, she said, the kind of place where you knew all your neighbors, never locked your doors, trusted everyone. The man who lived next door was a deacon at her church, very upstanding and respectable. One rainy day when she was five years old, he found her playing dolls in her family's garage. He closed the door, lifted up her dress, and rubbed his hand very hard against her groin. She didn't really understand what he was doing, but she knew from the strange look on his face that it was wrong, perhaps very naughty of her to let him, even though he hadn't asked her permission.

After he left, she felt dirty, as if she'd done something horribly wrong. Because she couldn't stop feeling bad about it, she decided to tell her mother.

"You're a liar!" her mother yelled and slapped her hard across the face. "He would never do such a thing!"

But Evelyn knew she was telling the truth, and when he touched her a second time, she learned to stay out of his way so it never happened again. Nevertheless, she was convinced that she must be a very bad girl for her mother to have reacted as she had, and she felt shamed and dirty.

When she got to high school and boys started asking her out, she almost never said yes. Or if she did, she wouldn't feel comfortable on a date until she'd had a couple of beers. Sometimes she would let a boy "fool around" with her, because she figured, what difference did it make? She was already contaminated. She was seventeen and about to graduate from high school when she decided to broach the subject again with her mother. Her mother's reaction was even more difficult to comprehend now that she was almost an adult. "It never happened," her mother declared. Then she forbade her to ever again bring up the subject.

That was when Evelyn got serious about drinking. "I drank so that at least for a little while I didn't feel evil or disgusting," she said. "I had a lot of bad relationships with men but I never married any of them. I never got involved with one man I could trust."

It took some doing, but I finally persuaded Evelyn to let me help her explore the source of her pain through a combination of sound, meditation, and visualization. Suddenly, she was feeling enormous rage toward her mother for having denied her reality and for putting the onus of shame on her, instead of where it properly belonged. For the first time in her life, she acted on her realization that she needed to be in therapy.

With a patient like Evelyn, who was consumed with guilt and anger, sound can be an extraordinary adjunct to psychotherapy. As we continued to work together, she reported to me that she was having bad dreams and not sleeping well. She was also feeling very irritable and cranky, and crying a lot. I asked her to think about the little girl who'd experienced that distrust. What did that feeling sound like? What was the sound of her guilt? And what about her rage?

She let out a low whimper, the sound of a little girl's cry, not even a groan. Then I asked her to contemplate her life song. I played the bowl for her, and we chanted the *bija* mantras together. Then I led her through a visualization as she thought about the sounds of her pain, and how they could be transformed by the ESSENCE meditation.

The change that came over her as she traversed the levels of consciousness described by Wilber was patently visible. That was the day she stopped drinking. Ultimately, she was able to experience emotional and spiritual healing as well as recovery from her alcoholism.

Evelyn's journey to wellness illustrates that healing transformation is well within our grasp. We do not have to travel to a mountain peak in a faraway country and sit in silent meditation in order to achieve peace and unity within our essence. We need only to use sound, meditation, and other modalities of the heart, so that we may hear what Larry Dossey describes as "the music of the body."

I imagine a time when Era III medicine will include these sound modalities:

- The use of crystal bowls and other instruments in group interventions for patients with life-threatening illness and chronic disease, both for psychospiritual development and physiologic entrainment.

- The widespread implementation of sound and music interventions for improved surgical outcomes, pain management, immune enhancement, cardiovascular fitness, and the treatment of mood disorders.

- The acceptance among healthcare personnel of the role of voice in healing, with training for nurses and physicians in the basic techniques of toning and singing for emotional expression, release, creativity, and healing.

- The broad application of the principles and practices of music thanatology in hospitals and hospices, to bring countless patients comfort and serenity as they go through the dying process.

- Commitment on the part of the medical community to research on the molecular and energetic correlates, and consequences, of sound and music healing modalities on the body's organs, tissues, cells, and DNA.

It is my fervent hope, of course, that mainstream medicine, already on a path toward greater acceptance of complementary medical approaches, will work toward these goals, funding research and implementing sound and music modalities in clinics and hospitals around the country. But realistically, I know that such developments will primarily be spurred by patients, the medical consumers who are beginning to recognize, from their own experience and intuition, that sound and music are extraordinarily powerful healing tools. I am certain that the humanization of medicine, which has been largely though not exclusively a patient-driven phenomenon, will soon encompass sound and music. Indeed, as Helen Bonny so eloquently put it, "As medicine moves toward holistic approaches that integrate body, mind, and emotion, it becomes more like music, which has always concerned itself with a person's total beingness."

When the day arrives that sound and music are fully integrated elements of a technologically superior yet humane medicine, then doctors and patients, working together, will be able to release the soaring potentialities of the human spirit.

# Bibliography

Achterberg, Jeanne. *Imagery in Healing.* Boston: New Science Library Shambhala, 1985.

Achterberg, J., B. Dossey, and L. Kolkmeier, *Rituals of Healing.* New York: Bantam Books, 1994.

Andrews, Ted. *Sacred Sounds: Transformation through Music & Word.* St. Paul, Minn.: 1996.

Beaulieu, John. *Music and Sound in the Healing Arts.* Barrytown, N.Y.: Station Hill Press, 1987.

Benson, Herbert, M.D. *The Relaxation Response.* New York: Avon, 1975.

Bentov, Itzhak. *Stalking the Wild Pendulum.* Rochester, Vt.: Destiny Books, 1988.

Berendt, Joachim-Ernst. *The World Is Sound: Nada Brahma.* Rochester, Vt.: Destiny Books, 1987.

Borysenko, Joan, Ph.D. *Minding the Body, Mending the Mind.* New York: Bantam Books, 1988.

Brodie, Renee. *The Healing Tones of Crystal Bowls.* Vancouver, B.C: Aroma Art Ltd., 1996.

Bush, Carol. *Healing Imagery and Music.* Portland, Ore.: Rudra Press, 1995.

Campbell, Don. *The Mozart Effect.* New York: Avon Books, 1997.

———. *The Roar of Silence.* Wheaton, Ill.: The Theosophical Publishing House, 1989.

Campbell, Don, ed. *Music: Physician for Times to Come.* Wheaton, Ill.: Quest Books, 1991.

———. *Music and Miracles.* Wheaton, Ill.: Quest Books, 1992.

Dossey, Larry, M.D. *Healing Words: The Power of Prayer and the Practice of Medicine.* New York: HarperCollins, 1993.

———. *Recovering the Soul.* New York: Bantam, 1989.

Dreher, Henry. *The Immune Power Personality.* New York: Dutton, 1995.

Feuerstein, Georg. *The Shambhala Guide to Yoga.* Boston: Shambhala Publications, 1996.

Gardner, Kay. *Sounding the Inner Landscape.* Rockport, Mass.: Element Books, 1990.

Gardner-Gordon, Joy. *The Healing Voice.* Freedom, Calif.: The Crossing Press, 1993.

Garfield, Laeh Maggie. *Sound Medicine: Healing with Music, Voice, and Song.* Berkeley, Calif.: Celestial Arts, 1987.

Gaynor, Mitchell L., H.D., and Jerry Hickey, R.Ph. *Dr. Gaynor's Cancer Prevention Program.* New York: Kensington Books, 1999.

Gaynor, Mitchell L., M.D. *Healing Essence: A Cancer Doctor's Practical Program for Hope and Recovery.* New York: Kodansha, 1995.

Gerber, Richard, M.D. *Vibrational Medicine.* Santa Fe, N.M.: Bear & Company, 1988.

Goldman, Jonathan. *Healing Sounds.* Rockport, Mass.: Element Books, 1992.

Goleman, Daniel, and Joel Gurin, eds. *Mind/Body Medicine: How to Use Your Mind for Better Health.* Yonkers, N.Y.: Consumer Reports Books, 1993.

Halpern, Steven, with Louis Savary. *Sound Health: The Music and Sounds that Make Us Whole.* San Francisco: Harper & Row, 1985.

Harner, Michael. *The Way of the Shaman.* San Francisco: HarperCollins: 1990.

Jansen, Eva Rudy. *Singing Bowls: A Practical Handbook of Instruction and Use.* Diever, Holland: Binkey Kok Publications, 1990.

Judith, Anodea. *Wheels of Life.* St. Paul, Minn.: Llewellyn Publications, 1995.

Kabat-Zinn, Jon. *Full Catastrophe Living.* New York: Delacorte Press, 1990.

———. *Wherever You Go, There You Are.* New York: Hyperion Books, 1994.

Katsh, Shelley, and Carol Merle-Fishman. *The Music Within You.* Gilsum, N.H.: Barcelona Publishers, 1998.

Keyes, Laurel Elizabeth. *Toning: The Creative Power of the Voice.* Marina del Rey, Calif.: DeVorss and Co., 1973.

Khan, Hazrat Inayat. *The Music of Life.* New Lebanon, N.Y.: Omega Publications, 1988.

Lerner, Michael. *Choices in Healing.* Boston: The MIT Press, 1994.

Levine, Stephen. *Guided Meditations, Explorations, and Healings.* New York: Anchor Books, 1991.

————. *Healing into Life and Death.* Garden City, N.Y.: Anchor Press, 1987.

Locke, Steven, M.D., and Douglas Colligan. *The Healer Within: The New Medicine of Mind and Body.* New York: New American Library, 1986.

Madaule, Paul. *When Listening Comes Alive.* Norval, Ontario: Moulin Publishing, 1994.

Maman, Fabien. *The Role of Music in the Twenty-first Century.* Redondo Beach, Calif.: Tama-Do Press, 1997.

Maranto, Cheryl Dileo, ed. *Music Therapy: International Perspectives.* Pipersville, Pa.: Jeffrey Books, 1993.

McClellan, Randall. *The Healing Forces of Music.* Rockport, Mass.: Element Books.

Moyers, Bill. *Healing and the Mind.* New York: Doubleday, 1993.

Naparstek, Belleruth. *Your Sixth Sense.* San Francisco: Harper San Francisco, 1997.

Newham, Paul. *The Singing Cure.* Boston: Shambhala, 1993.

Pert, Candace B., Ph.D. *Molecules of Emotion: Why You Feel the Way You Feel.* New York: Scribner, 1997.

Rider, Mark. *The Rhythmic Language of Health and Disease.* St. Louis: MMB Music, 1997.

Rossman, Martin L. *Healing Yourself.* New York: Pocket Books, 1987.

Saionji, Masami. *Infinite Happiness: Discovering Your Inner Wisdom.* Rockport, Mass.: Element Books, 1996.

Schwartz, Tony. *What Really Matters.* New York: Bantam Books, 1995.

Siegel, Bernie. *Love, Medicine & Miracles.* New York: Harper & Row, 1986.

Simonton, O. Carl., Stephanie Matthews-Simonton and James L. Creighton. *Getting Well Again.* New York: Bantam Books, 1992.

Spintge, R., M.D., and R. Droh, M.D., eds. *MusicMedicine.* St. Louis: MMB Music, 1992.

Tomatis, Alfred A. *The Conscious Ear.* Barrytown, N.Y.: Station Hill Press, 1991.

# Recommended Resources

## Sound, Music, and Guided Imagery

Mitchell Gaynor, M.D.
*The Gaynor-Hickey Health Report*
Phillips Publishing, Inc.
7811 Montrose Road
Potomac, Maryland 20854-3394
Telephone: (800) 777-2002
*A monthly newsletter devoted to integrative healing and a plan for disease-free living, providing the latest in nutritional supplements and aids for meditation, including ESSENCE guided imagery tapes, Tibetan and crystal bowls.*

The Venerable Shyalpa Rinpoche
Ranrig Yeshe Center
P.O. Box 1167
Stockbridge, Massachusetts 01262
Telephone: (413) 528-9932
E-mail: mhlafrance@earthlink.net
*For information and instruction in Tibetan and Dzogchen meditation practices.*

Belleruth Naparstek
Image Paths, Inc.
891 Moe Drive, Suite C
Akron, Ohio 44310-2538
Telephone: (800) 800-8661
Fax: (330) 633-3778
E-mail: hjtapes@aol.com
Website: www.healthjourneys.com
*For information about Naparstek's speaking schedule, to order imagery tapes, or to receive* Health Journeys Network News.

Linda Rodgers
Audio Prescriptives Foundation
70 Maple Avenue
Katonah, New York 10536
Telephone: (914) 232-6405
*To order tapes designed to alleviate anxiety before, during, and after surgery, using guided imagery, calming music, and suggestions.*

Jonathan Goldman
Sound Healers Association
P.O. Box 2240
Boulder, Colorado 80306
*For information on sound-related seminars and workshops.*

Steven Halpern
Inner Peace Music
P.O. Box 2644
San Anselmo, California 94979
Telephone: (415) 485-5321
Fax: (415) 485-1312
E-mail: innerpeacemusic@innerpeacemusic.com
Website: www.innerpeacemusic.com
*To order Steven Halpern's CDs, cassettes, videos and CD-ROMs.*

MMB Music, Inc.
Contemporary Arts Building
3526 Washington Avenue
St. Louis, Missouri 63103
Telephone: (314) 531-9635, (800) 543-3771 (United States/Canada)
Fax: (314) 531-8384
E-mail: mmbmusic@mmbmusic.com
Website: www.mmbmusic.com
*Excellent source for books on music, sound, and healing.*

Jim Oliver
Oliver Music
P.O. Box 6508
Santa Fe, New Mexico 87502-6508
Telephone: (505) 466-9991
Fax: (505) 466-9992
E-mail: jomusic@compuserve.com
*To order CDs and tapes composed and orchestrated by Oliver to promote relaxation and healing.*

Jeffrey Thompson, M.D.
Brain/Mind Research
204 N. El Camino Real, E116
Encinitas, California 92024
Telephone/Fax: (800) 349-7358
Website: www.body-mind.com
*For more information about Dr. Thompson's research and to order tapes.*

## For information about GIM therapists and training

Association for Music and Imagery
Attn: James Rankin
331 Soquel Avenue, Suite 201
Santa Cruz, California 95062

The Bonny Foundation
2020 Simmons Street
Salinas, Kansas 67401

Mid-Atlantic Institute
Attn: Carol A. Bush
Box 4655
Virginia Beach, Virginia 23454
Telephone: (757) 498-0452

## Sound, Music, Healing, and Medicine

Don Campbell, Inc.
The Mozart Effect Resource Center
P.O. Box 4179
Boulder, Colorado 80306
Telephone: (800) 721-2177
*For information on seminars, workshops, and classes by Campbell, and to order books and tapes.*

Chalice of Repose Project
Therese Schroeder-Sheker, Coordinator
School of Music Thanatology
554 West Broadway
Missoula, Montana 59802
*For information about services to the dying, as well as music-thanatology training program at St. Patrick's Hospital in Missoula.*

International Society for Music in Medicine
Ralph Spintge, Director
Sportkrankenhaus Hellerson
Paulmannshoher Strasse 17
D5880 Ludenscheild, Germany
*International organization for research, meetings, and publishing.*


The Open Ear Center
Pat Moffitt Cook, Director
6717 N.E. Marshall
Bainbridge Island, Washington 98110
Telephone: (206) 842-5560
*For information about courses, seminars, and resources for music and healing.*


SoulSongs
Shulamit Elson
The Center for Sound Healing
P.O. Box 465
High Falls, New York 12440
Telephone: (914) 687-7783, (212) 714-4611
E-mail: soulsongs@aol.com
Website: www.soulsongs.com
*For information about workshops, retreats, and healing circles that focus on toning and healing.*


Jill Purce
Healing Voice
20 Willow Road
Hampstead, London NW3 1TJ
England

Telephone: 0171-794-9841

Fax: 0171-435-4331

Website: www.jillpurce.com

*For information about how to order Purce's tapes and books, as well as schedule of workshops on overtone chanting, sonic meditation, and other sound-related topics.*

Tama-Do

Attn: Christina Ross

The Academy of Sound, Color, and Movement

22937 Arlington Avenue, #203

Torrance, California 90501

*For information about Fabien Maman's healing and sound workshops in the United States and France.*

Tree-of-Life Mystery School

Joseph-Mark Cohen, Director

TLMS, Box 1355

Ainsworth, British Columbia V0G 1A0

Canada

Telephone: (800) 775-0712, X 3777 (between 3 and 5 P.M., PST)

E-mail: jm-cohen@netidea.com

*For information about workshops on sound and Kabbalistic healing, harmonics, meditation, and movement, as well as to order video- and audiotapes on these and other subjects.*

**For information about the Tomatis method**

The Listening Centre, Tomatis Canada

Paul Madaule, Director

599 Markham Street

Toronto, Ontario M6G 2L7

Telephone: (416) 588-4136

Sound Listening and Learning Center, Tomatis USA
Billie Thompson, Ph.D., Director
2701 E. Camelback, Suite 205
Phoenix, Arizona 85016
Telephone: (602) 381-0086

Tomatis International Headquarters
Christian Tomatis, Director
144 Avenue des Champs Elysées
Paris 75008, France
Telephone: 01 53 53 42 40

## Music Therapy

The American Music Therapy Association
8455 Colesville Road, Suite 1000
Silver Spring, Maryland 20910
Telephone: (301) 589-3300
Fax: (301) 589-5175
E-mail: info@musictherapy.org
Website: www.musictherapy.org

The Certification Board for Music Therapists
589 Southlake Boulevard
Richmond, Virginia 23236-3093
Telephone: (800) 765-2268, (804) 379-9497
Fax: (804) 379-9354

The World Federation of Music Therapists, Inc.
P.O. Box 585
01080
Vitoria-Gafteiz, Spain
Telephone: 3445-143-311
Fax: 3445-144-224

# Notes

## 1. SOUND ESSENCE

30    "The Popul Vuh": David MacLagan, *Creation Myths* (London: Thames & Hudson, 1977), p. 30.

30    The Athabascan tribe: Merlin Stone, *Ancient Mirrors of Womanhood: Our Goddess and Heroine Heritage*, vol. 2 (New York: New Sibylline Books, 1979), p. 97.

30    According to the Hopis: MacLagan, *Creation Myths*, p. 30.

31    In Navajo mythology: Jamake Highwater, *Ritual of the Wind* (New York: Viking Press, 1977), p. 17.

31    For Native Americans: Highwater, ibid., p. 36.

31    Bruce Chatwin, in his splendid book: Bruce Chatwin, *The Songlines* (New York: Penguin Books, 1987), p. 13.

31    "[They] . . . wandered over the continent. . . .": ibid., p. 2.

31    The Hindu tradition traces its origins: Georg Feuerstein, *The Shambhala Guide to Yoga* (Boston: Shambhala Publications, 1996), pp. 98–104.

33    Singing is a form of communication: Yehudi Menuhin and Curtis W. N. Davis, *The Music of Man* (New York: Simon & Schuster, 1979), p. 7.

34    Eskimos of eastern Greenland: Edmund Carpenter, *I Breathe a New Song: Poems of the Eskimo*, ed. Richard Lewis (New York: Simon & Schuster, 1971), p. 22.

34    The tribeswomen of New Guinea: Steven Feld, *Sound and Sentiment* (Philadelphia: University of Pennsylvania Press, 1982), p. 33.

34    In ancient Greece: Randall McClellan, *The Healing Forces of Music* (Rockport, Mass.: Element Books, 1991), p. 5.

34    The story is told: ibid.

34    The Apaches: Penelope Washburn, ed., *Seasons of Women* (San Francisco: Harper & Row, 1979), p. 15.

34    Women in Finland: ibid., p. 54.

34    Among the Pueblos: ibid., p. 104.

34    In East Africa: David Meltzer, ed., *Birth: An Anthology of Ancient Texts, Songs, Prayers, and Stories* (San Francisco: North Point Press, 1981), p. 215.

36    In his seminal book, *The Way of the Shaman:* Michael Harner, *The Way of the Shaman* (San Francisco: HarperCollins, 1990), p. 51.

37    Neher theorized: ibid., p. 52.

37    Research conducted by Wolfgang Jilek: ibid.

40    One Kabbalistic source, the *Sefer Bahir:* Edward Hoffman, *The Way of Splendor: Jewish Mysticism and Modern Psychology* (Northvale, N.J.: Jason Aronson, 1992), p. 156.

41    The thirteenth-century *Zohar:* ibid., p. 157.

42    My ideas about well-being: Hazrat Inayat Khan, *The Music of Life* (New Lebanon, N.Y.: Omega Publications, 1988), p. 261.

42    As summarized by Steven Locke, M.D.: Steven Locke and Douglas Colligan, *The Healer Within: The New Medicine of Mind and Body* (New York: New American Library, 1986), pp. 14–15.

43    In the words of Hazrat Inayat Khan: Khan, *The Music of Life,* p. 6.

43    According to Inayat Khan: ibid., p. 25.

43    Inayat Khan eloquently articulated this idea: ibid., p. 27.

45    "They discovered ways . . . of shaping their vocal cavities": Jonathan Goldman, *Healing Sounds* (Rockport, Mass.: Element Books, 1992), p. 66.

49    As I searched for information on the subject: Joachim-Ernst Berendt, *The World Is Sound: Nada Brahma* (Rochester, Vt.: Destiny Books, 1987), p. xi.

50    "We ourselves are rhythm . . .": Khan, *The Music of Life,* p. 12.

## 2. FLOATING IN THE BEAUTY

53    Among the most notable was . . . Claude Bernard: Henry Dreher, *The Immune Power Personality* (New York: Dutton, 1995), p. 19.

53    Bernard's work was further developed: ibid., p. 20.

54    All of these conditions: Locke, and Colligan, *The Healer Within,* p. 15.

54    all of our various biological systems are connected: Dreher, *The Immune Power Personality,* p. 14.

55    But the interactions that reveal: Candace B. Pert, Ph.D., Henry E. Dreher, and Michael R. Ruff, Ph.D., "The Psychosomatic Network: Foundations of Mind-Body Medicine," *Alternative Therapies in Health and Medicine,* vol. 4, no. 4 (July 1998): 30.

67    Think back to Huygens's observation: Berendt, *The World Is Sound,* p. 116.

68    Brian L. Partridge . . . has said: ibid., p. 118.

68    Referring specifically to this predilection: ibid., p. 119.

68    Consider this extraordinary example: ibid., p. 117.

69    Rudolf Haase, a German musicologist: ibid., p. 119.

69    Other forms of entrainment: ibid., p. 117.

70    Condon filmed many conversations: Anodea Judith, *Wheels of Life* (St. Paul: Llewellyn Publications, 1995), p. 286.

70    "Listeners were observed to move . . .": W. S. Condon, *Journal for Autism and Childhood Schizophrenia,* 5:1 (1975): 43.

70    "Synchronized heartbeats have been reported . . .": Berendt, *The World Is Sound,* p. 118.

70    Research over the past two decades: Jonathan S. Goldman, "Sonic Entrainment," in *Music—Physician for Times to Come,* ed. Don Campbell (Wheaton, Ill.: Quest Books, 1991), p. 221.

72    Siegel cites a study: Bernie Siegel, *Love, Medicine & Miracles* (New York: Harper & Row, 1986), p. 37.

74    Jeanne Achterberg cites an analysis: Jeanne Achterberg, *Imagery in Healing* (Boston: New Science Library Shambhala, 1985), p. 44.

75    Researchers Stephen Garret and Daniel Statnekov: Goldman, "Sonic Entrainment," p. 229.

75    "Our ability to *have* a world": George Leonard, *The Silent Pulse* (New York: E. P. Dutton, 1978), p. 18.

## 3. THE POWER OF MUSIC AND VOICE

77    Joseph Moreno, a music therapist: Joseph J. Moreno, "The music therapist: creative arts therapist and contemporary shaman," in *Music—Physician for Times to Come*, p. 167.

78    "Being in harmony with oneself . . .": Steven Halpern with Louis Savary, *Sound Health: The Music and Sounds that Make Us Whole* (San Francisco: Harper & Row, 1985), p. 39.

78    During a 1956 visit with Tilly: William McGuire and R. F. C. Hull, eds., *C. G. Jung Speaking: Interviews and Encounters* (Bollingen Series XCVII, Princeton, N.J.: Princeton University Press, 1977), pp. 273–275.

79    Guzzetta has explored: B. Dossey, L. Keegan, C. Guzzetta and L. Kolkmeier, *Holistic Nursing: A Handbook for Practice* (Aspen, Colo.: Aspen Publishers, 1988), pp. 263–288.

80    Reduced anxiety, heart and respiratory rates: J. M. White, "Music therapy: an intervention to reduce anxiety in the myocardial infarction patient," *Clinical Nursing Specialties*, 6:2 (1992): 58–63.

80    Reduced cardiac complications: C. E. Guzzetta, "The effects of relaxation and music therapy on patients in a coronary care unit with presumptive acute M.I." *Heart and Lung*, 18:6 (1989): 609.

80    Lowered blood pressure: Olav Skille, "Vibroacoustic Research 1980–1991," in *MusicMedicine*, ed. Ralph Spintge and R. Droh (St. Louis: MMB Music, 1991), p. 249.

81    Reduced blood pressure and heart rate: Tony Wigram, "The Psychological and Physiological Effects of Low Frequency Sound and Music," *Music Therapy Perspectives*, 13 (1995): 16–35.

81    Blood pressure and excessive noise: Bill Gottlieb, ed., "Sound Therapy," *New Choices in Natural Healing* (Emmaus, P.A.: Rodale Press, 1995), p. 126.

81    Reduced blood pressure, heart rate, and noise sensitivity: J. F. Byers and K. A. Smyth, "Effect of a music intervention on noise annoyance, heart rate, and blood pressure in cardiac surgery patients," *American Journal of Critical Care*, 6:3 (1997): 183–191.

81    Increased immune cell messengers: Dale Bartlett, Donald Kaufman, and Roger Smeltekop, "The effects of music listening and perceived sensory experiences on the immune system as measured by interleukin-1 and cortisol," *Journal of Music Therapy*, 30 (1993): 194–209.

82    Drop in stress hormones during medical testing: J. Escher, et al. [Music during gastroscopy} {German]. *Schweiz. Med. Wochenschrift*, 123 (1993): 1354–1358.

82    Boost in natural opiates: "Music/Endorphin Link," *Brain/Mind Bulletin* (Jan. 21 and Feb. 11, 1985): 1–3.

83 "... music therapy ranks high on the list": Arthur W. Harvey, "Music in Attitudinal Medicine," in Campbell, *Music—Physician for Times to Come*, p. 189.

83 "half an hour of music ...": quoted on the Music for Healing and Tansition Program website at www.vashonisland.com/MHTP.

83 Anesthesiologist Ralph Spintge, M.D.: Ralph Spintge, "Music as a Physiotherapeutic and Emotional Means in Medicine," *Musik, Tanz und Kunst Therapie* 2/3 (1988): 79.

84 Harvey paid a visit: Campbell, *Music—Physician for Times to Come*, p. 186.

84 A similar perspective: interview, Nov. 12, 1998; Linda Rodgers, "Music for Surgery," *Advances*, 11:3 (1995): 49–57.

85 One recent clinical trial: Henry Dreher, "Mind-body interventions for surgery: evidence and exigency," *Advances*, 14:3 (1998): 207–222.

87 "For people who have motor problems ...": Evelyn Gilbert, "Musical Medicine," *Village Voice*, Sept. 2, 1997, p. 45.

87 At a 1991 Senate special committee meeting: hearing before the Senate Special Committee on Aging, "Forever Young: Music and Aging," U.S. Senate, Aug. 1, 1991, reported in *Music Therapy Perspectives*, 10 (1992): 59–60.

88 Clarkson reports the case of Jerry: Ginger Clarkson, "Adapting a Guided Imagery and Music Series for a Nonverbal Man with Autism," *Association for Music and Imagery Journal* (1995): 123–137.

89 Fifty percent of women: R. Droh and Ralph Spintge, *Anxiety, Pain, and Music in Anesthesia* (Basel: Roche Editions, 1983).

89 A group of women in Vancouver, Canada: Carlos E. Gonzalez, "The music therapy-assisted childbirth program: a study evaluation," *Pre- & Peri-Natal Psychology Journal*, 4:2 (1989): 111–124.

89 periods of music alternating with periods of silence: Suzanne B. Hanser, Sharon C. Larson, and Audree S. O'Connell, "The effect of music on relaxation of expectant mothers during labor," *Journal of Music Therapy*, 20:2 (1983): 50–58.

89 Research conducted with infants: Jacquelyn Michele Coleman, Rosalie Rebollo Pratt, Ronald A. Stoddard, et al., "The effects of the male and female singing and speaking voices on selected physiological and behavioral measures of premature infants in the intensive care unit," *International Journal of Arts Medicine*, 5:2 (1997): 4–11.

90 In a Tallahassee, Florida, hospital: Keith Caine, "The effects of music on the selected stress behaviors, weight, caloric and formula intake, and length of hospital stay of premature and low birth weight neonates in a newborn intensive care unit," *Journal of Music Therapy*, 28 (1991): 180–192.

90 Schroeder-Sheker stumbled upon her calling: Therese Schroeder-Sheker, "Music for the dying: A personal account of the new field of music thanatology—history, theories, and clinical narratives," *Advances*, 9:1 (1993): 36–48.

92 "The fetus hears an entire range ...": Alfred A. Tomatis, *The Conscious Ear* (Barrytown, N.Y.: Station Hill Press, 1991), p. 127.

92 "By his very structure ...": ibid., p. 125.

93 As part of his research: ibid., p. 127.

93 "I do not treat children": ibid., p. 45.

93 To bring clients: Paul Madaule, *When Listening Comes Alive* (Norval, Ont.: Moulin Publishing, 1994), p. 36.

94    According to Paul Madaule: ibid., p. 60.

94    This phenomenon led Tomatis to conclude: ibid., p. 34.

94    Tomatis offers this answer: Tomatis, *The Conscious Ear*, p. 160.

95    . . . Campbell cites research: Campbell, *The Mozart Effect*, p. 15.

95    In his book *Pourquoi Mozart*: ibid., p. 27.

95    "Alana and her twelve-year-old daughter": Joy Gardner-Gordon, *The Healing Voice* (Freedom: Calif.: The Crossing Press, 1993), pp. 100–101.

97    "Toning is an ancient method . . .": Goldman, *Healing Sounds*, p. 136.

97    "Toning is a system of healing . . .": Garfield, p. 57.

97    "Tone is simply an audible sound": Don G. Campbell, *The Roar of Silence* (Wheaton, Ill.: The Theosophical Publishing House, 1989), p. 62.

97    "Toning is the process of making vocal sounds": John Beaulieu, *Music and Sound in the Healing Arts* (Barrytown, N.Y.: Station Hill Press, 1987), p. 115.

97    Toning is "the sustained vocalization": McClellan, op. cit.

97    "Toning is an activity": Steven Halpern, *Tuning the Human Instrument* (Belmont, Calif.: Spectrum Research Institute, 1978), p. 169.

98    "Toning is the use of the voice": Goldman, *Healing Sounds*, p. 136.

98    On page 99 are simple directions: Gordon, op.cit., pp. 67–69.

99    See the adapted versions: ibid., pp. 108–109.

101    "Anyone can use toning": Campbell, *The Mozart Effect*, p. 92.

101    Keyes described the sense of exhilaration: Laurel Elizabeth Keyes, *Toning: The Creative Power of the Voice* (Marina del Rey, California: DeVorss and Co., 1973) pp. 12–13.

101    According to Hazrat Inayat Khan: Khan, *The Music of Life*, pp. 274–275.

101    Lisa Sokolov . . . believes that voice: Shelley Katsh and Carol Merle-Fishman, *The Music Within You* (Gilsum, N.H.: Barcelona Publishers, 1998), p. 152.

102    Here are two exercises: ibid., pp. 152–154.

103    She describes the latter: Pythia Peay, "Singing the Soul Home," *Common Boundary*, July/August 1998, p. 24.

#### 4. GOOD VIBRATIONS

110    When Soos asked what he could do: Eva Rudy Jansen, *Singing Bowls: A Practical Handbook of Instruction and Use* (Diever, Holland: Binkey Kok Publications, 1990), p. 5.

111    In the words of Tibetan monk: Mitch Nur, *Sacred Metals of Tibet*, pamphlet compiled for Sacred Sounds Workshop Retreat, October 1997, p. 10.

113    According to one legend of Atlantis: Renee Brodie, *The Healing Tones of Crystal Bowls* (Vancouver, B.C.: Aroma Art, 1996), p. 18.

114    When electric current is applied: Richard Gerber, M.D., *Vibrational Medicine* (Santa Fe, N.M.: Bear & Company, 1988), p. 337.

114    "The crystalline structure . . .": ibid., p. 338.

115    As Michael Harner explains: Harner, *The Way of the Shaman*, p. 109.

115    Marcel Vogel, who worked as a senior scientist: Gerber, *Vibrational Medicine*, p. 338.

115    As Gerber points out: ibid.

### 5. SOUND BODY

133    Dr. Greer and his colleagues showed: S. Greer, K. W. Pettingale, T. Morris, et. al., "Mental attitudes to cancer: an additional prognostic factor," *Lancet*, 1 (1990): 49–50.

134    "The physical effect of sound . . .": Khan, *The Music of Life*, p. 269.

135    Candace Pert has pointed out: Pert et al., "The Psychosomatic Network."

135    Walleczek has proven: J. Walleczek and R. P. Liburdy, "Nonthermal 60Hz sinusoidal magnetic-field exposure enhances 45Ca2+ uptake in rat thymocytes: dependence on mitogen activation," *FEBS Letter*, Oct. 1, 1990 (271, 1–2): 157–160; J. Walleczek, "Electromagnetic field effects on cells of the immune system: the role of calcium signaling," *FASEB Journal*, 6:13 (1992): 3177–3185; J. Walleczek and T. F. Budinger, "Pulsed magnetic field effects on calcium signaling in lymphocytes: dependence on cell status and field intensity," *FEBS Letter*, Dec. 21, 1992 (314–3): 351–355.

136    Maman's dual interest: Fabien Maman, *The Role of Music in the Twenty-first Century* (Redondo Beach, Calif.: Tama-Do Press, 1997), pp. 45–46.

136    Maman found that the most visibly dramatic results: ibid., pp. 59–61.

136    Based upon his findings: Don Campbell, *The Mozart Effect* (New York: Avon Books, 1997), p. 243.

137    "This finding indicates . . .": Maman, *The Role of Music*, pp. 117–118.

137    Maman also collaborated: ibid., p. 61.

138    I was especially fascinated to learn: Kay Gardner, *Sounding the Inner Landscape* (Rockport, Mass.: Element Books, 1990), p. 120.

139    Sir Peter Guy Manners . . . has researched and developed: compiled by Burton Goldberg Group, *Alternative Medicine* (Fife, Wash.: Future Medicine Publisher, 1994), p. 446.

139    Manners views disease: Gardner, *Sounding the Inner Landscape*, p. 125.

139    "By intercepting the electrical messages . . .": Goldberg, ibid., *Alternative Medicine*, p. 446.

139    Cymatic therapy . . . has been used to treat: Gardner, *Sounding the Inner Landscape*, p. 126.

139    Manners hopes: Goldberg, *Alternative Medicine*, p. 446.

140    Thompson creates an acoustical mix: Jeffrey Thompson, D.C., interview, May 27, 1997.

141    Thompson believes that this similarity: ibid.

143    Potanin finds the blending: Con Potanin, M.D., interview, May 25, 1997.

143    a group of university students was lectured: Mark S. Rider and Cathy Weldin, "Imagery, improvisation, and immunity," *Arts in Psychotherapy* 17:3 (1990): 211–216.

144    In another experiment: M. S. Rider, J. Achterberg, G. E. Lawlis, et al., "Effect of immune system imagery on secretory IgA," *Biofeedback and Self-Regulation*, 15:4 (1990): 317–333.

144    Rider and Achterberg carried out a study: M. S. Rider and J. Achterberg, "Effect of music-assisted imagery on neutrophils and lymphocytes," *Biofeedback and Self-Regulation*, 14:3 (1989): 247–257.

144    "Amazingly, only the blood cell [type] . . .": Rider, *The Rhythmic Language of Health and Disease*, p. 130.

144    Pioneering work conducted in the mid-'70s: J. Achterberg, G. E. Lawlis, O. C. Simonton, et al., "Psychological factors and blood chemistries as disease outcome predictors for cancer patients," *Multivariate Experimental Clinical Research*, 3 (1977): 107–122.

145 an increase in natural killer cell activity: R. Zachariae, J. S. Kristensen, P. Hokland, et al., "Effect of psychological intervention in the form of relaxation and guided imagery on cellular immune function in normal healthy subjects," *Psychotherapy and Psychosomatics*, 54 (1990): 32–39.

145 increased production of IgA: M. L. Jasnoski and J. Kugler, "Relaxation, imagery, and neuroimmunomodulation," *Annals of the New York Academy of Sciences*, 496 (1987): 722–730.

146 significantly greater activity and numbers: H. Hall, "Hypnosis and the immune system: A review with implications for cancer and the psychology of healing," *American Journal of Clinical Hypnosis*, 25 (1983): 92–103.

146 selective boosting or dampening: G.R. Smith, J.M. McKenzie, D.J. Marmer, et al, "Psychologic modulation of the human immune response to varicella zoster," *Archives of Internal Medicine*, 145 (1985): 2110–2112.

150 Jeanne Achterberg eloquently describes: Jeanne Achterberg, *Imagery in Healing*, pp. 19–20.

150 During the Middle Ages: Therese Schroeder-Sheker, "Music for the dying: A personal account of the new field of music thanatology—history, theories, and clinical narratives," *Advances*, 9:1 (1993): 36–48.

## 6. SOUND FEELINGS

160 He was astonished to discover: Herbert Benson, M.D. and Eileen M. Stuart, R.N., M.S., *The Wellness Book* (New York: Birch Lane Press, 1992), p. 35.

161 In one study of twelve shift-working nurses: Mark S. Rider, Joe W. Floyd, and Jay Kirkpatrick, "The effect of music, imagery, and relaxation on adrenal corticosteroids and the re-entrainment of circadian rhythms," *Journal of Music Therapy*, 22 (Spring 1985): 46–58.

162 An enterprising group of Japanese researchers: Y. Satoh, H. Nagao, H. Ishihara, et al., "An objective evaluation of anxiolytic effect of music for surgical patients," *Masui: Japanese Journal of Anesthesiology*, 32 (10), (1983): 1206–1211.

162 As Mark Rider points out: Mark Rider, *The Rhythmic Language of Health and Disease* (St. Louis: MMB Music, 1997), p. 106.

168 Research has shown that even in utero: Lee Salk, M.D., "Mother's Beat as an Imprinting Stimulus," in R. O. Benezon, ed., *Music Therapy Manual* (Springfield, Ill.: Charles C. Thomas, 1981).

168 Dr. Thomas Verny . . . describes studies: Dr. Thomas Verny, *The Secret Life of the Unborn Child* (New York: Dell, 1981).

178 As with the ritual uses of sound: Rider, *The Rhythmic Language*, p. 187.

178 "Eventually, the cacophony drowns out . . .": ibid.

## 7. SOUND SPIRIT

183 As Ram Dass has written: Ram Dass, "Relative Realities," in Roger N. Walsh and Frances Vaughn, *Beyond Ego: Transpersonal Dimensions in Psychology* (Los Angeles: Jeremy P. Tarcher, 1980), p. 139.

190  According to Daniel Reid: Daniel Reid, *The Complete Book of Chinese Health and Healing* (Boston: Shambhala Publications, 1994), p. 293.

## 8. EXPLORING THE INNER CHAMBER

207  Belleruth Naparstek describes a phenomenon: Belleruth Naparstek, *Your Sixth Sense* (San Francisco: Harper San Francisco, 1997), p. xiv.

207  "opening my *heart* to this other person": ibid., p. xviii.

211  The Japanese word for "intuition": Masami Saionji, *Infinite Happiness: Discovering Your Inner Wisdom* (Rockport, Mass.: Element Books, 1996), pp. 24–25.

213  In their own research, the Greens: Tony Schwartz, *What Really Matters* (New York: Bantam Books, 1995), pp. 148–149.

213  such highly respected . . . intuitives: Naparstek, *Your Sixth Sense*, p. 41.

214  "We actually inhabit a universe . . .": ibid., pp. 100–101.

216  Bentov described a theory of solid matter: Itzhak Bentov, *Stalking the Wild Pendulum* (Rochester, Vt.: Destiny Books, 1988).

216  "Our body is the pendulum": Naparstek, *Your Sixth Sense*, p. 104.

219  As a small child, Jill Purce: Jill Purce, "The Healing Voice," brochure published by Inner Sound, London, England.

221  a moving example of the power of GIM: Sara Jane Stokes, "Letting the Sound Depths Arise," in *Music and Miracles*, compiled by Don Campbell (Wheaton, Ill.: Quest Books, 1992), p. 194.

222  the ultimate objective of GIM: Carol Bush, *Healing Imagery and Music* (Portland, Ore.: Rudra Press, 1995), p. 84.

222  Bush suggests the exercise: ibid., pp. 187–205.

226  this simple, meditative reflection: Saionji, *Infinite Happiness*, p. 30.

## 9. SOUND SYNTHESIS

227  Larry Dossey, M.D., describes what he calls: Larry Dossey, M.D., *Recovering the Soul* (New York: Bantam, 1989).

232  as Helen Bonny so eloquently put it: Helen Bonny, Ph.D., "Music and Healing," *Music Therapy*, 6A:1 (1986), p. 6.

# Index